A Tangled Web

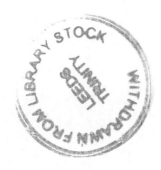

New International Studies in Applied Ethics

VOLUME I

EDITED BY

Professor R. John Elford,
Leeds Metropolitan University

EDITORIAL BOARD

Professor Simon Lee, Vice-Chancellor of Leeds Metropolitan University

Professor Charles E. Curran, Elizabeth Scurlock Professor of Human Values,
Southern Methodist University in Dallas

Professor Celia Deane-Drummond, Chester University

Professor Heidi Hadsell, Professor of Social Ethics
and President of Hartford Seminary

The Very Revd Ian S. Markham, Dean of Virginia Theological Seminary

Professor Keith Ward, Regius Professor of Divinity, Emeritus, University of Oxford

PETER LANG

Oxford · Bern · Berlin · Bruxelles · Frankfurt am Main · New York · Wien

A Tangled Web

Medicine and Theology in Dialogue

R. John Elford and D. Gareth Jones (eds)

PETER LANG

Oxford · Bern · Berlin · Bruxelles · Frankfurt am Main · New York · Wien

Bibliographic information published by Die Deutsche Bibliothek
Die Deutsche Bibliothek lists this publication in the Deutsche National-
bibliografie; detailed bibliographic data is available on the Internet at
<http://dnb.ddb.de>.

A catalogue record for this book is available from The British Library.

Library of Congress Cataloging-in-Publication Data

A tangled web: medicine and theology in dialogue / edited by R. John
Elford and D. Gareth Jones.
    p. cm. -- (New international studies in applied ethics ; v. 1)
    Includes bibliographical references and indexes.
    ISBN 978-3-03911-541-9 (alk. paper)
    1. Medicine--Religious aspects--Christianity. 2. Medical ethics. I.
Elford, R. John. II. Jones, D. Gareth (David Gareth), 1940-
    BT732.T36 2008
    261.5'61--dc22

                    2008038947

© Peter Lang AG, International Academic Publishers, Bern 2009
Hochfeldstrasse 32, Postfach 746, CH-3000 Bern 9, Switzerland
info@peterlang.com, www.peterlang.com, www.peterlang.net

Printed in Germany

Contents

6

R. JOHN ELFORD

Preface

The book was prompted by visits by D. Gareth Jones to Liverpool, where a colloquium was held in April 2006. This was attended by most of the contributors to the volume, and some others. Papers were circulated beforehand and discussed. These have subsequently been modified and updated, and are now incorporated as chapters within this volume, whilst other chapters have been added.

The overall aim has been to explore the ways in which medical research and practice and Christian ethics can work together to their mutual benefit. This is an attempt to avoid the all too familiar antagonisms which so often feature elsewhere in this engagement. None of this, of course, avoids controversy and for that reason alone the debates will undoubtedly continue. If this volume helps to introduce into that process some positive areas of collaborative support, it will have succeeded in its purpose.

The areas chosen for discussion are, of necessity, selective: many more that require attention will occur to the reader throughout, and a sequel volume is in preparation. The final section, on Regulation and Policy, is included in order that the more theological and philosophical discussions might be related to actual practice. In this way, the book can be read as an essay in applied ethics. It is, in fact, the first in a forthcoming series of such books from Peter Lang entitled *New International Studies in Applied Ethics*, which will be based at Leeds Metropolitan University with me as general editor.

My co-editor and I sincerely thank all the contributors and those others who have been involved in the debates. We also thank Professor Simon Lee, Vice-Chancellor of Leeds Metropolitan University, for encouragement and financial support, Ms Val Fairfield, the typesetter, and Mr Alfred Westwell, the copy editor and proofreader.

D. GARETH JONES

Introduction

One of the frequent complaints made about scientific developments in biology and medicine is that they are outstripping the ability of our ethical systems to cope with them. If only it were possible to call a halt to these developments, to stop them for a while, so that our ethical systems could 'catch up', this would enable us to decide which developments are acceptable and should be allowed to continue, and which are not and should be banned. We are repeatedly told that we are playing God, overreaching ourselves, and attempting to accomplish things that should never be attempted. Without restraints to put an end to such endeavours, it is feared that some of the recent scientific developments will have far-reaching negative repercussions for the human race, since they will change for ever our own view of what we are as human beings. In other words, they will have profound philosophical and social implications.

Inherent within such responses is the strong desire that we should rein in scientists, since science is not an island unto itself. The activities of scientists, it is argued, are not simply of interest to an elite and privileged group of iconoclasts. All of us are affected, and probably in detrimental ways. The social context within which the biomedical sciences are carried out is of considerable interest to societies as a whole, and the direction these sciences take should be under the control of those societies. Perhaps this is a fair demand, but what might it mean and could it ever be a realistic goal?

General as these considerations are, their relevance for theology is clear. They present a challenge to theologians by asking what specific contributions theological perspectives might be able to offer to this ongoing debate. Such perspectives are urgently needed, since the questions being raised are, in the final analysis, theological in nature. For instance, the biomedical sciences force us to ask what it is that constitutes the core of humanness. Does this reside solely in biological characteristics, such as the organisation of our brains? Or is it much broader, encompassing our awareness of our place in the universe, our dependence upon a higher authority, our relationships with others in community, and our responsibilities for the ecosystem and other living things? These considerations, in turn, raise the question of human control. How much should human beings seek to control their world, including themselves, and how much should they accept will never be under human control, and perhaps never should be? How far should human beings go in modifying the way in which individuals function, or in determining the kind of children we wish to produce?

This question becomes even more urgent when the individuals concerned are not ill, and where the aim is to enhance them in some nebulous fashion. Is the prospect of improving human beings through biological modification to be welcomed or rejected? Theoretical as such a prospect still is at the present time, it is a matter for serious current debate in the reproductive realm, with the availability of pre-implantation genetic diagnosis (PGD) and the choice this opens up of selecting one embryo over another. There is no doubt that this is a consideration for bioethics, but is it also one for theology? Should the prospect of selecting one embryo over another, let alone that of far more radical biological modification, be anathema to those with a faith perspective, on the grounds that it is outside the domain of legitimate human activity? Is this exclusively God's realm, and if so on what basis? This is where bioethics and theology meet. Each is grappling with questions of startling novelty, and neither has the luxury of unlimited time to emerge with definitive solutions.

Bioethics and theology need not be in conflict, one dominating the other, but rather should be in dialogue. We shall achieve more when we recognise the value of what each discipline has to contribute to informed discussion of the issues raised by the progress of science. Dialogue is essential when the matters at hand are novel and intensely challenging. Also implicit within dialogue is an acceptance that definitive answers might not be attainable. Indeed, they may not even be desirable, since tentativeness and a willingness to adapt to unexpected findings and directions may be crucial.

However, statements like this immediately raise core concerns for some theologians and people of faith, because they appear to necessitate an abandonment of some of the essentials of their faith. These essentials may include the God-givenness of human beings in their present biological condition, or the sacredness of all human life from fertilisation onwards. Consequently, any biological development that entails interfering with human life gives the impression, perhaps inadvertently, of challenging these essentials. Intrusions are being made into divine territory. Bioethical debate that ignores this dimension is readily interpreted as antithetical to theological aspirations. Is this because certainty is being replaced by uncertainty and clear moral guideposts by vague and relative ones? Is contemporary bioethics too ready to permit all new scientific developments, thereby relinquishing any moral authority to draw lines in the sand?

Concerns of this sort are understandable, and have to be taken very seriously. The quandary is to know how best to address them. And this is where the writings in this book have a role to play. Though they are selective in the topics chosen, leaving many areas unaddressed, they touch on aspects of some of the fundamental debates at the contemporary interface of bioethics and theology. While we as contributors acknowledge that we raise more questions than we can answer, it is our hope that we will provide pointers that will prove beneficial in future discussions.

This book is the product of collaboration between medical and theological writers, and it is hoped that this will enrich the discussion rather than prove a distraction. While the theologians reflect on what they recognise as central theological themes and considerations raised by scientific endeavours, I write as a scientist working within the Christian tradition.

This subdivision of tasks mirrors the way in which much of the general bioethical debate is conducted within society. Scientists are at the forefront of the developments, and many wish to know the potential significance of what it is they are doing. While some may speak with unnerving assurance about the good that will almost inevitably (they think) emanate from their work, the majority are far more circumspect. They want guidance about the implications of what they are undertaking. They are not unaware of moral imperatives, even though they may have little expertise in how to think ethically: their expertise is in laboratory science, not in ethical or philosophical thinking. Perhaps it should be otherwise; perhaps scientists should have to undergo basic ethical training. However, even if that were to eventuate (and it is unlikely), they would remain little more than amateur participants in highly demanding territory. That would be unsatisfactory: far better to have vigorous dialogue between various experts who respect one another's contributions.

While as contributors we accept the limitations of each of our disciplinary perspectives, we are firmly committed to interdisciplinary dialogue. We need to listen to one another, just as all theologians, bioethicists and scientists need to. We have much to learn by doing so, but this inevitably involves humility and an openness that may be foreign to each of us.

The problems confronting us are formidable. Too often it is the voices of the most outspoken that get heard, regardless of whether these represent mainstream opinion or a minority viewpoint. This situation is exacerbated by the role of the media in influencing public perception: the controversial, the novel and the extreme make better stories than the moderate and seriously considered. Furthermore, it is far too easy to rely on information in the form of simplistic soundbites expecting yes/no, agree/disagree responses. None of this makes for profitable dialogue.

Taken together these responses feed the public imagination, which in the area of health is intimately linked to finding instant cures for incurable conditions. The slightest whiff of a scientific break-through readily translates into a cure for a serious condition tomorrow, or at least the day after. This by itself is highly problematic, and is made even more so by claims of cures by practitioners (generally in unregulated regimes) based upon unsubstantiated work that has not been assessed in an appropriately rigorous manner. Sometimes the claims are based on outright fraud. The consequences for patients and their families can be devastating. Resorting to these forms of experimental treatment might be fuelled by compassion, and yet it is a compassion that lacks an ethical base. Unhelpful and misleading treatment regimes are profoundly deceptive and destructive of hope, regardless of how much they purport to be based on compassion. Once more, we find ourselves in territory familiar to theologians, with its emphasis upon those values that will best uphold the interests of people.

How, then, are theologians to think about the issues raised by advances in biomedical science? Neither the Bible nor Christian tradition directly addresses many of the particulars of the pertinent issues. How could they? Until recent times, no one had conceived of the present technologies, least of all any of the biblical writers, Church Fathers, or Reformers. What they have provided us with are general principles and directions, and it is these we have to come to grips with in this arena. The grandeur and fallenness of human beings, the centrality of human community and relationships, the dignity and value of human beings as those created in the image and likeness of God, constitute crucial bioethical imperatives. The *imago Dei* is frequently cited in bioethical discussions, but it brings with it two apparently polar concepts: a respect for the existing design of creation and the human attribute of creativity. As bioethicists and theologians enter into dialogue with each other, it will be against a backdrop of considerations such as these.

It is interesting to note, however, that this dialogue does not take place between two well-defined positions. While the technologies that underpin contemporary medicine are certainly novel, both the bioethical and theological responses are also far from well established. It is inevitable that theological responses are not fully pre-formed, but rather develop in response to issues as they arise. Our ability to foresee future possibilities in science (and perhaps in many other spheres of human activity) has been woefully inadequate, leading to an inability to formulate refined positions in advance. It is as if both the bioethical and theological approaches are struggling to find how best to respond. Which are the most applicable fundamental values to use, and how are these to be determined?

In his chapter, R. John Elford focuses on the priority of love. Yet within this he points out that even when this principle has been embraced, the loving course of action in a particular situation is not necessarily clear. Although there may be agreement on the Christian principles that we consider as best applying to a specific bioethical quandary, there might still be intense disagreement about the nature of the resultant Christian standpoint to be taken on that issue.

Any adequate Christian response to bioethical issues also has to take account of its effect on actual people, including those in our churches, our families and even ourselves. This is the pastoral dimension to bioethical decision making. We need to formulate responses that are practical, accessible and compassionate towards the struggles of real people. Difficult decisions have to be made by infertile couples, the parents of sick children, the children of ageing parents, and those with terminal conditions, as well as by scientists, clinicians, moral philosophers and moral theologians. The context of so many of these decisions is that of suffering. The pastoral domain reminds us that neat solutions are rarely to be found, decisions so often being tainted with uneasy compromise. Nevertheless, such dimensions have to be taken into account when dialogue takes place between bioethics and theology.

The chapters of this book also bring us face-to-face with the vocabulary we employ to describe the perceived influence of newly emerging technologies on populations and patients. Myriad examples abound, only a few of which are touched on here. These include 'eugenics' in connection with PGD, and 'enhancement' when dealing with radically idealised extensions of clinical therapeutic interventions. Such notions – eugenics and enhancement in this case – carry fearful connotations, ensuring that the clinical procedures associated with them will likely be rejected. As long as these concepts remain unexplored, there is no apparent need to tackle the issues arising from currently available clinical procedures. Acting in this manner, however, is destructive of serious bioethical assessment, just as it is of serious theological analysis. By ignoring the potential contributions of both, all subsequent debate becomes be seriously undervalued.

Discussion on all these issues is frequently intertwined with legal and regulatory considerations, to the extent that these sometimes colour the whole debate. Important as these considerations are, their role in ethical and theological discussion should be carefully assessed. The connection between legal and ethical approaches is far from straightforward. On the one hand, there is a tendency in some quarters to look to legal regulations to solve what are fundamental social and moral (and perhaps theological) problems. On the other hand, when legal regulations are at the behest of changing social forces and mores, they can be notoriously fickle. The coherence between ethics (let alone theology) and the law is often flimsy and ephemeral, as is demonstrated in later chapters. One of the lessons to emerge is that changing social attitudes, as much as developing scientific findings, are responsible for prompting the modification of regulatory stances. The question that inevitably follows is: what influence, if any, might theology have in such cases?

How to respond to regulatory processes is, in fact, one of the most difficult areas for theologians. As the chapters in Part Three demonstrate, it is far easier to critique these processes than to find a way of contributing to society-wide discussions. This is partly due to the highly problematic nature of public consultation, which is prone to being manipulated in one direction or another, and partly also to the inherent difficulty of expecting nuanced responses to highly complex issues. An all-too-clear example of these problems is provided by the current debate in the UK on allowing the creation of human admixed embryos, namely, cybrids (cytoplasmic hybrid embryos) or chimeras. The public face of the debate is that of a science/religion divide, with scientists intent on finding cures for as yet incurable diseases and theologians aghast at the grotesqueness and Frankenstein overtones of these possibilities. The choices presented by this divide are stark and unwelcome, since the theological desire to protect human dignity and human life is equated with a lack of concern for patient welfare. Distracting as all this is, the absence of scientifically informed discussion is woeful, and serious questions about the relationship between the human and non-human in developing cybrids and the meaning of species boundaries in chimeras remain unaddressed. It is tragic that little room is being made for interdisciplinary scientific, philosophical and theological analysis. This is one area where a huge amount of work is required to discern the best way in which theological voices can be heard. The contrast here between the UK and the US contexts is stark, since theological voices appear to have little scope in the former but extensive scope in the latter. However, in practice the differences in the two societies are far less obvious, since regulation in the USA applies to the public federal sphere, leaving the private sphere relatively uncontrolled. A fitting topic for another col-loquium and book will be how theology and Christian spokespeople can contribute to, and enter more effectively into, the public debate over regulation. A start, and hopefully a useful one, has been made in this volume.

Part One: Theological Background

GERARD MANNION

Theologically-Informed Ethics:
A New (Old) Paradigm?

Introduction

The stereotypical picture of the Christian contribution to debate about advances in our understanding of what it is to be human and how we might enhance human being, above all through the rapid developments in genetic science, frequently portrays the churches as offering conservative and backward-looking perspectives that serve simply to hamper 'development' and 'advancement'. Of course, some Christian approaches to ethical issues have not helped matters here. Some have sought to lecture the 'world without' that they perceive to be 'beyond' the church and to offer the Christian narrative and 'tradition' (understood in the singular) as *the only* solution to the contemporary ills of the world. This volume does not entertain such an approach. It is concerned rather with seeking an approach whereby Christian voices in pluralist societies are neither rubbished nor ignored, but instead are recognised as being able to make genuine and yet no less critical or less informed contribution to the pressing moral debates of the times. This chapter explores some methodological and background issues about how such interdisciplinary conversations and dialogue might prosper.

Some ten years ago, the Anglican moral theologian Nigel Biggar identified one of the most pressing questions for Christian moral and ecclesial reflection today:

> ... given the dramatic fall in church membership since the Second World War, and given the growth in public responsibility and popularity of alternative religious and non-religious beliefs, it is not clear what moral authority Christian churches can reasonably be expected to wield nowadays. Perhaps the churches

have been speaking; it's just that non-Christians haven't been listening. And why should they? Were it the case that the morality espoused by the churches is peculiarly Christian in all its aspects, were it the case that it made sense only on the basis of peculiarly Christian beliefs about God, then it could have little relevance or appeal to non-Christians. But this is not so. Christian morals do not depend at every point and entirely on Christian faith. Nor is all the content of Christian faith exclusively Christian.[1]

Indeed, the question can be broadened further still – has the Christian church anything to say of value, with regards to morality, to a post-modern, increasingly relativistic and/or nihilistic world today? Has it any right to do so? Or should its primary concern be with the discourse and practice of morals *within* the bounds of its own community? Many people today continue to believe that the church can, should and must play such a role vis-à-vis the wider world community,[2] but that it should do so in a dialogical and collaborative fashion with other groups, traditions and communities, both religious and secular. Indeed, they argue that Christians will need to adapt and modify aspects of Christianity's moral traditions along the way, to enable its adherents to confront the changing moral dilemmas and contexts of differing times and different places.

And yet Christians who wish to offer something to ethical discourse and to make positive contributions to moral discernment about contemporary dilemmas beyond the confines of their own particular religious communities are faced with an especially problematic situation today. They have to meet the daunting task of trying to steer their open and developing approach to ethics between two threatening perils. On one side, the Scylla of a world increasingly sceptical, not simply about morality in general, but also about religion and religious values in particular. Vehement secular voices see religion as illusory (or, as Dawkins has recently famously put it, delusional), irrelevant and even harmful and pernicious. The other dangerous obstacle is the

1   Nigel Biggar, *Good Life: Reflections on What We Value Today* (London: SPCK, 1997), p.133, cf. also p.135. A related discussion can be found in Keith Ward, *Religion and Community* (Oxford: OUP, 2000), pp.228–33.
2   See James M. Gustafson, *Ethics from a Theocentric Perspective*, vol. 2, *Ethics and Theology* (Chicago: Chicago University Press), p.317.

Charybdis of a growing retreat from the world by the many Christians who believe the postmodern era to be so full of threats to their community and way of life that the best course of action is to turn away from the evils of the sinful world and focus in upon their own community and values so as to avoid further 'infection' from the harmful vices and temptations of secular modernity and now post-modernity.

The middle course of navigation, which seeks to allow Christianity today to offer something of lasting value to the wider world and the moral dilemmas that beset it, to engage in dialogue with that world so that Christianity can both give and receive in such encounters, is captured well by the vision espoused by Frank Kirkpatrick:

> If postmodern ethics is looking to preserve the pluralism of human life, it can do no better than to look to a theistic ethic in which 'remarkably and gloriously complex' forms of humanity are manifested, but always under the guiding intention of bringing persons to their fullest possible flourishing in and through mutual love.[3]

In this chapter I wish to make a case for renewed and expanded dialogue across disciplines with regard to moral dilemmas and ethical discourse in general. I want to suggest reasons why what Frank Kirk-patrick says here can be embraced as insightful, indeed even true, by non-Christian scientists, as much as it can be by pluralistic-minded Christians themselves. In other chapters, hopefully, we shall see the proof of the pudding that such an approach might yield.

My essential thesis, then, is that ethics need not be perceived as something which must be kept 'pure', untainted by the influence of non-religious worldviews and value systems. Nor even do particular religious worldviews and value systems have a monopoly on moral truth. So, for example, I would consider as misguided the approach taken by those Christians who turn inwards and suggest that they must attend primarily to their own community and its way of being, who think that their value system is the only ultimately true one and that

---

3   Frank G. Kirkpatrick, *A Moral Ontology for a Theistic Ethic: Gathering the Nations in Love and Justice* (Harmondsworth: Ashgate, 2003), p.147.

other approaches to moral dilemmas must always fall short of the attainment of moral truth.

Instead, I wish to make a case for theologically-*informed* ethics: ethical discourse and insights that can be enhanced through what theological enquiry and reflection can bring to the table. One need not be of a particular religious persuasion, disposition or conviction to learn from, and gain moral insight through, such theologically-informed ethical discourse. Similarly, this is an approach which recognises the value of other moral approaches and ethical methods as well; ones which are informed by differing worldviews and outlooks. The end result is greater conversation and dialogue across the disciplines, within and between cultures and a process of mutual learning between differing contexts.[4]

Thinking about 'Rights' and 'Wrongs' from a Christian Perspective: The Communitarian Dimension of Morals and the Moral Dimension of Community

In discerning the nature, scope, and history of Christian moral discourse, we are confronted with questions of a fundamentally ontological nature. Christians profess faith in a God who is a community of persons, and the realisation of the will and purpose of that God in this world and in the lives of all humans who are called to respond to the gracious offer of that God's self-communication forms the basis of the Christian perspective of the 'good life', and hence of Christian moral discourse. Here social ontology and self-realisation coincide. There is no conflict between upholding the inherent dignity of every human person and continuing to hold fast to the supreme importance

---

4   This would be contrary to the recent arguments of, say, Gavin D'Costa, who
     would appear to privilege anew theology and even to afford it disciplinary pre-
     eminence, but who departs from his otherwise critical engagement with the
     disciplines when he discusses theology itself, and particularly when discussing
     official church pronouncements.

of community. One contemporary specialist in the ethics of community, Frank Kirkpatrick, champions a *relational* moral ontology as the basis of a theistic ethic,[5] perceiving mutuality geared towards full human flourishing as being 'the necessary ontological foundation on which a theistic religious community must be built'.[6] The Christian ideal of community is therefore bound up with the Christian idea of morality.

Elsewhere in this volume, Gareth Jones illustrates how sometimes certain scientists put individual choices and needs above the wider social and community interests. Theologically-informed ethics can be particularly helpful in ensuring that a better balance is maintained between research and regulation.

Christians and Morality: Re-envisioning the Interaction

We thus further contemplate the intricacies of some contemporary ecclesiological questions in moral and social ontology. Regardless of the differing ecclesial and ecclesiological schools of thought here, the important questions that preoccupy much of their contemporary dis-

---

5   Kirkpatrick also observes (*A Moral Ontology*, p.123) how this point is made in the work of Karl Rahner: 'There is an *individuum ineffabile* that cannot be overridden by general moral principles. Persona and community are, in short, "correlative"; as persons we are intended for community with God and other persons, and real community exists only where our nature as persons is protected.' There is no ultimate paradox between communion and uniqueness. The Rahner citation in Kirkpatrick is taken from Gustafson, *Ethics and Theology*, pp.76–77. See, also, Kirkpatrick, *A Moral Ontology*, p.146: '... community is the context of flourishing and flourishing serves the mutuality that constitutes community. As Eric Loewy observes, without community, personal freedom and fulfilment are meaningless concepts. "Community is the necessary condition of freedom and fulfilment, the soil in which individual life is rooted and without which is inevitably dies".' Here Kirkpatrick is citing Loewy, *Suffering and the Beneficent Community* (Albany: State University of New York Press), p.xvi.
6   Kirkpatrick, *A Moral Ontology*, p.148.

cussion are fundamentally the same. They include: what is the nature of the church's relationship to the wider world, and hence what is the nature of the role which the church is called to play in that world? What is the task for Christian ethicists, and what *sort* of ethics should they be shaping and writing about? What form of moral discourse and formation is most appropriate, both within the confines of the church itself and with regard to the true relation of the church to the world? Do the answers to such questions depend, ultimately, upon our understanding of the nature of the church's very being and the moral dimension of such being, in other words, upon what social and moral ontologies we adhere to and by which we shape our discourse and praxis?

Here, we will explore such questions by examining, first, what is meant by the very notion of the church as a *moral* community. Next we shall revisit certain fluctuations in Christian moral discourse throughout the last century or so, thereby providing some background to the contemporary debates concerning the relationship between the church and morality. This will enable us to focus attention upon what I wish to suggest has become (once again) the fundamental issue of focus in recent debates, namely, the relationship between the church, its members and the world 'beyond' the confines of the church. In doing so, we shall explore how certain thinkers believe that our views concerning the church/world relationship have an overriding impact upon both our ecclesiological and our ethical thinking and practice.

Christianity and the Idea of a Moral Community

So, the church constitutes a 'moral community' – a community engaged in moral discernment.[7] What does it mean to conceive of the church as such? Furthermore, in speaking of the ethics of the Christian community, what might be said of the twofold sense of this term: that

7   For a denominationally comparative and inter-faith discussion of this ecclesial conception, see Ward, *Religion and Community*, chapter 9.

is, the morals by which a community is shaped and organised, as well as the *form* of moral discernment and the resultant moral principle by which the community lives?

The importance of exploring the relationship between the church and morality is underscored by James Gustafson, on the fundamental need for, and importance of, 'communities of moral discourse':[8]

> The importance of [moral] communities cannot be overstressed. Even significant choices made by individuals in problematic circumstances are more likely to 'value right' the good or evil before them if opportunities for reflection and consultation occur in the presence of another person. When more complex matters of public policy ... are under consideration a community is indispensable. ... no single person has the capabilities to be sufficiently informed about factual matters, analyses or processes and patterns of inter-dependence, and projection of possible consequences of alternative courses of action to be absolutely self-reliant. ... Discernment ought to be a social as well as individual process.[9]

I wish to broaden this notion: scientists and legislators, along with numerous other 'players' in public life today, can all form part of a wider 'community of moral discourse', a community that listens to all voices and which privileges no particular interest group save the vulnerable.

Here space prevents us revisiting the debates about whether or not there is such a thing as 'Christian ethics', as well as those concerning the differences between 'moral theology' and 'Christian ethics' and the like, although elements of that debate will be touched upon as the argument progresses.

The upheavals of the twentieth century, and the perpetual developments in different traditions and in the way in which people do theology and ethics, have led to profound changes in the differing ways in which Christians engage in moral discernment. Thus, by the second half of the last century, Protestant Christians would engage with and learn from the methods of moral theology, and Roman

8   Gustafson develops the arguments put forth in an earlier work of his: 'The Church: A Community of Moral Discourse', in *The Church as Moral Decision Maker* (Philadelphia: Pilgrim Press, 1970), pp.83–95.

9   Gustafson, *Ethics and Theology*, pp.184, 316.

Catholics, in line with the profound changes that the mid-late twentieth century witnessed in Catholic theology in general (as well as in the church itself), began to see a broader scope for moral discernment. So, for example, this allowed for a re-emphasis on the importance of the Bible as a source for guidance in people's lives and also led to many Catholic moral theologians stressing the importance of the *lived experience* of Catholics, illustrating how this could and should inform the church's own moral teaching.

Perhaps the greatest change was that historical consciousness and contextual considerations began to influence how Christians engaged in ethical discernment. In Catholic approaches in particular, ethical methods had previously been based upon an approach that perceived the world in 'organic' terms, as a whole that could be readily understood as such (and thus moral discernment was seen as a process of *deduction* from generalities in order to identify responses to specific dilemmas). Gradually, there came a realisation of the pressing need to discern the 'signs of the times' and an understanding that different contexts and geographical and social, not to mention existential, situations called for a more nuanced approach in moral matters (rather than universal and absolute principles being applied in the same way in all places and at all times). Thus, approaches became more *inductive*: reasoning from specifics and only then seeking to shape more general principles and norms. Though, as we shall see, older ways of thinking did persist in many quarters and actually became increasingly influential in repristinated forms throughout the church in the closing decades of the last century and into the present. But, by the late twentieth century, for many people the terms 'Christian ethics' and 'moral theology' had become interchangeable.[10]

---

10   See the textbooks such as Hamel and Himes and also that edited by Bernard Hoose, *Christian Ethics: An Introduction*, which draw no distinction between the two.

How, Where and When Christians Engage in Moral Discourse

The arena of debate surrounding Christian ethics and moral theology has, in recent decades, become one where much confusion has reigned, but also one where a new and intense polarisation between differing schools of thought has emerged – and this perhaps in response to the blurring of the distinctions, not simply between the two approaches but also between Christian and 'secular' ethics, such as philosophical ethics, political and social theory and so on, not to mention the approaches to ethics found in other faiths. In other words, broader debates about how Christians should perceive the relationship between their community, their church and the wider world have had a profound impact upon how Christians have sought to understand the processes of moral discernment in a postmodern age, where new and intense moral dilemmas present themselves before Christians and challenge traditional moral norms and values in so many different ways. For the purposes of this volume, we obviously see that human advancement and developments in genetic science pose new and increasingly complex challenges for Christian moral discourse.

It is thus in this sense that renewed debates have emerged in relation to how one understands what it is to be a Christian and what it is for a community to be a church impacts significantly upon how one understands the processes of moral discernment.

Many Christians had begun to try and transcend a 'particularist' approach to doing ethics, rediscovering perhaps something of the fundamental benefit of not simply natural law reasoning, but also of character and virtue-based moral reasoning (which transcends specific contexts, times, traditions and cultures, and is more transferable and indeed flexible in its application to differing and changing particular dilemmas and situations). But other Christians have felt that the churches and certain Christian ethicists have 'sold out' far too much to modernity and liberalism and have allowed the essentials of Christian moral norms and values to become watered down. Hence some argue for a restoration of the emphasis upon the *distinctiveness* of Christian

norms and values. Still others have called for an abandonment of the
notion that Christians 'do ethics' altogether. Rather, they suggest,
Christians should concentrate on being 'church', and all the right
moral pathways might follow from attention to doing so. The secular
world needs ethics, their argument goes, but Christians just need to be
Christian.

So, as an example of the first type, consider the recent constructive perspectives offered by Christoph Baumgartner,[11] who, despite
equating Catholic moral theology and 'theological ethics', is none the
less correct in charting the development of moral theology as a separate discipline from the end of the sixteenth century onwards.[12] He
recognises, also, the contemporary difficulties that we have identified
here, and suggests that they have come about because moral theology
has, ever since that era, 'Developed in a way that has led to a situation
which is distinctly different from its origin', namely from the context
of confessional practice to today when, 'in the light of the Christian
understanding of the world and of all humanity, [it] reflects on the
right and proper behaviour of all human life'.[13] As such, moral theology now requires an 'interdisciplinary methodology'.

Baumgartner thus reflects upon the various changes that the
discipline has undergone, including its nomenclature, and charts a
tendency for theological ethics to become 'institutionally independent
within the canon of theological disciplines'.[14] He admits this is likewise true for other sub-disciplines within theology and is perhaps best
understood in the growing prevalence of specialisation in numerous
'sciences'. But the question that many Christians have raised in the
light of such developments is whether this has led to the 'detheologisation' of ethics – whereby the theological component of moral
theology is taken as read and is regarded as not requiring particular
elucidation and explanation.[15]

11   Christoph Baumgartner, 'Theological Ethics Without Theology', in *Theology in
     a World of Secularisation*, ed. Erik Borgman and Felix Wilfred, *Concilium* 2,
     2006, pp.53–64.
12   Ibid., p.53.
13   Ibid.
14   Ibid., p.54.
15   Ibid.

Baumgartner defines ethics as 'the academic reflection of human behaviour and action, of moral norms, attitudes and views, as well as of social institutions from the perspective of what is good and right'.[16] *Theological* ethics is thus an undertaking from 'within the Christian understanding of the world and of human beings'.[17]

Baumgartner's own attempt to answer the questions he poses begins with the assertion that theology, by definition, must move with the times. Furthermore, because there are so many forms of ethics, in one sense talk of a specific theological ethics 'is impossible'.[18] Thus the 'detheologisation' thesis would be rejected because ethics is always a wider undertaking and theological approaches are always attentive to the broader cultural and intellectual currents of a given time and context. On the other hand, we do see complications arise in the case of some schools of thought where certain ethical concepts are explicitly developed within the context of theology – and he cites liberation theology and the work of Emmanuel Levinas as two prime examples.

Nonetheless, within the framework of ideological pluralism in liberal societies, the answers to the questions surrounding the 'detheologisation' thesis are not so clear cut. Christianity claims that its message is 'for all people' which, Baumgartner argues, implies that its 'insights are *discovered*, in the light of the Christian view of the world and [therefore] its people cannot form a "specifically religious morality"'.[19] The ethical norms that entail obligation must be applicable to all, and hence require 'argumentative foundations beyond the boundaries of specific groups or communities of faith'.[20] Thus theological convictions, logically speaking, cannot provide the main force of argument in moral discourse, as non-Christians would not share them.

Does this mean that theological ethics becomes indistinguishable from philosophical ethics and now simply dances to the same liberal tune? In Baumgartner's opinion, the answer is a resounding 'no', for

---

16   Ibid., p.56.
17   Ibid.
18   Ibid.
19   Ibid., p.58.
20   Ibid.

such a conclusion would actually overlook the distinction between ethics of *obligation* and an ethics of *ambition*, with fundamental methodological differences pertaining between the two.[21] He explains this by suggesting that the former explores questions about what is 'just' and the latter about what is 'good'.[22]

We will explore some of these debates in a touch more detail. But the first problem might be further illustrated if we explore the broad consensus which Christians from numerous different denominational backgrounds settled upon in the latter years of the twentieth century. This, broadly speaking, led to the transcending of the old divides and to reference to the interchangeability of moral theology and Christian ethics. But a second approach that emerged − and perhaps (notwithstanding Baumgartner's reflections) a solution with more logical rigour than such a confusing compromise − was to speak of 'theological ethics'. In general, then, this refers to ethics that arise out of the theological sub-disciplines and which are fashioned with reference to the substance and ends of theological enquiry and Christian witness. But, even here, genuine and consistent methodological consensus has proved illusory (and here Baumgartner offers a convincing case in support).

The Church and the 'World'

Where the church has had a real dilemma and issue for debate from its very beginnings is the relationship between the church and the world, and the ecclesial attitudes and practices which relate to, shape and reflect this. Kirkpatrick frames the question in these terms:

---

21   Ibid., p.59.
22   Though he does acknowledge that the *specifically* theological forms of ethics cited above, for example liberation theology and Levinas's moral thought, must be treated differently.

The engagement of the church (more or less understood along *koinonia* lines) and the secular society is an issue that presently divides many Christian ethicists and theologians. This is not simply a question of what the proper relations between church and states ought to be. Underneath the legalities of church/state relations, there is the deeper, more fundamental question for any ethics of community of what attitudes and engagements between the ecclesia and society (sometimes limited to what is called the State) are theologically and morally justified. This is a more basic question in some ways than deciding which form of society (e.g., liberal or communitarian) is the most desirable from a Christian ethical point of view. Sometimes the question is posed as one of the relation simply between the church and the 'world'.[23]

In the second half of the last century, the World Council of Churches and the Second Vatican Council shifted the balance in ecclesial thinking towards more openness and engagement with the wider world. Here consider the mottos of many of the WCC's General Assemblies, or Vatican II's *Gaudium et Spes*, the Pastoral Constitution on the Church in the Modern World.

Ethics of a Christian Character and Christians who do Ethics – Revisiting another Old Debate

However, in many quarters of the Christian church, the balance has swung back in the other direction in recent years. Fears of secularisation along with a range of reactions to the 'postmodern situation' have caused many theologians, church leaders and, crucially, those engaged with the grass roots movements in various denominations, to turn 'inwards' once more; in other words (in sociological parlance) to perceive of the church as a *world-renouncing* as opposed to a *world-affirming* community. Let us explore the parameters of this debate further, for they have a marked bearing upon the involvement of Christians in contemporary moral discourse.

---

23   Frank G. Kirkpatrick, *The Ethics of Community* (Oxford: Blackwell, 2001), p.103.

Thus, the ethical writings of some Christians in recent decades have been concerned with championing anew, in one form or another, the distinctiveness of the moral discourse in which Christians engage, much as there has been a similar attempt to defend the distinctiveness of Christian theology from secular culture and to insist on its independence from, or even superiority to, other academic disciplines. Indeed, some figures question the validity of our speaking of any impartial discipline such as 'ethics' or even a sub-discipline such as 'Christian ethics' at all.

Theologically-Informed Ethics: A Christian–Secular Imperative?

We now return for more positive food for thought to Christoph Baumgartner, who explored the possibility of 'Theological Ethics Without *Theology*'. Contrary to the neo-exclusivists and the theologians who accentuate difference from the world, he believes that recent developments in moral theology do *not* constitute a detheologising (that is, a deficiency of overt theological emphasis) but rather 'should be perceived as a specific method which indeed enables theological ethics at all to make a contribution as theological ethics to solve the moral problems posed by free and liberal societies which are pluralistic in their world views'.[24] Hence, along similar lines to the argument I have been attempting to construct in this chapter, Baumgartner believes that in order for theology to fulfil its universal mission it must be obliged to respect 'relevant standards of science of each historical situation'.[25] This, of course, is of key relevance for the issues under consideration throughout this volume, and the chapters that follow demonstrate the validity of such an argument.

Thus, Baumgartner continues, contemporary methods will differ considerably from those, for example, of scholastic exegetes, not be-

---

24   Baumgartner, 'Theological Ethics Without Theology', p.60.
25   Ibid.

cause detheologisation has indeed triumphed but rather 'for the sake of the cause of Christianity', for, after all, theology is the 'science of faith'.[26] And such constitutes a 'necessary condition' in order for theology to make a contribution today at all.[27] Along similar lines, we see the noted social ethicist Judith Merkle suggest the following:

> Awareness of pluralism will help the Church find its place in the policy debate. Religious institutions in a democracy operate at the nexus of public opinion and public policy decisions. They rarely form decisions, rather they contribute to the framework that sets limits for policy choices and provides indications of policies desired by the public. For the Church to be effective in this role in a pluralistic society, it has to speak in terms that members of the public can understand. In order to be heard in the wider public debate, the Church needs to express values in non-religious terms so that other can find them morally persuasive.[28]

As Baumgartner concludes, sometimes theologians might not refer to God or the Christian faith explicitly, but nonetheless theological ethics is still a theological discipline. Indeed, for universal moral principles and norms this 'is methodologically appropriate'.[29]

If one sought to discern a concrete example of the vision of theologically-informed ethics as proposed and understood here, as well as of that lucid and insightful interpretation offered by Baumgartner, one would do well to try and capture, and to apply in a still broader context, something of the spirit of the following statement with which Lisa Sowle Cahill concluded her recent review essay on recent developments in theological bioethics:

> Theological bioethics should strive to reshape domestic and international health policy through political participation, as well as through the traditional venues of scholarship and education. Theologians addressing bioethics have an opportunity and a responsibility to redefine the social agenda of the field to highlight compassionate care and to favor the needs of the poor. The specific

---

26   Ibid.
27   Ibid., p.61.
28   Judith Merkle, *From the Heart of the Church* (Collegeville: Liturgical Press, 2004), p.253, drawing upon Bernadin's *A Moral Vision for America*, ed. John P. Langan SJ (Washington DC: Georgetown University Press, 1998), p.15.
29   Baumgartner, 'Theological Ethics Without Theology', p.61.

issues of death and dying highlight the inequality and deprivation that plague
access to health resources worldwide. To change this situation should be the
first priority of theological bioethics.[30]

Baumgartner reminds his readers of how John Rawls and, especially,
Jürgen Habermas (and to their names I would add that of Raymond
Plant) attempt to suggest constructive ways in which religious worldviews can come to play significant roles within liberal societies. Two
prerequisite conditions are necessary in order that they might do so.
The first is that universal norms must be justified in ways that everyone in the given society can accept. The second is that religions must
attempt to try and secure 'practical loyalty' to such universal norms
through embedding those norms within the respective religious worldviews.[31] Habermas argues (Baumgartner succinctly illustrates) that the
conceptions of the good informed by the worldviews mentioned in the
second condition will nonetheless need to be revised in the light of the
conception of 'the right', entailed by the first.[32]

Baumgartner thus concludes that theological ethics does indeed
fulfil such a task, since the function of theological ethics is actually,
on the one hand, to provide a 'critical evaluation of religion'[33] and, on
the other, 'to provide a critical perspective to universally held moral
norms'.[34] Hence the critique of *both* the inward-looking (community-
oriented) perspective and the outward-looking perspective (oriented
solely towards the wider world and concrete societal institutions) that
emerges may actually 'lead to a strengthening of the identity of theology' itself.[35] Amen to that.

---

30   Lisa Sowle Cahill, 'Notes on Moral Theology: Bioethics', *Theological Studies*
     67, 2006, p.142.
31   Baumgartner, 'Theological Ethics Without Theology', p.61.
32   Habermas's example here is the attitude towards homosexuals.
33   Here he utilises the thought of Alfons Auer.
34   Baumgartner, 'Theological Ethics Without Theology', p.61.
35   Ibid., p.62.

Conclusion

Many, many persons and numerous movements fought long and hard battles to recover the open and embracing communitarian vision of the gospel anew in the modern, and now postmodern, world. To do so, across the denominational divide, they fought against exclusivistic, sectarian and insular tendencies wherever they found them. Those battles were far too important and much too exhausting simply to permit exclusivism, in whatever form, to rear its ugly head again and dominate the ecclesial and ethical agenda for Christians in a new century. Nor should we entertain any notion of capitulating to the 'terrorism' and intellectual crudeness of the new fundamentalists – those aggressively atheistic and pathologically anti-religious scientists and philosophers, as well as media commentators who hog the airwaves, newsprint and popular bookshelves far too much these days.

Christians are thus today called to challenge ecclesial and moral perspectives that appear to reject any affirmation of the interwovenness of the secular and sacred in history, but rather must seek for an application of the monistic conception of history familiar to liberation theology, and indeed also inspired by thinkers such as Karl Rahner who tells us that 'there is no separate and sacral realm where God alone is to be found'. Augustine had particular contextual reasons for writing *The City of God* in the way that he did, but today we no longer need to explain the demise of the Roman Empire and so need no rigid demarcation of what is the religious and what is the secular – far better to be concerned with 'finding God in all things'.

Christians must not forget that the church, from its very beginnings, has always utilised, borrowed and learnt from 'secular' notions and models of authority and governance – sometimes to its detriment, often to its gain. (How else could it champion human rights and dignity today?) Too often we see demands for a somewhat unreflective biblicalist and simplistic pneumatological ecclesial agenda put up against more open and dialogical ecclesiologies. It is most ironic that here such demands overlook how littered with 'secular' socio-political themes the Bible actually is, and that the conceptualisation of the church's understanding of the doctrine of the Trinity draws heavily on secular socio-political and philosophical thought of bygone ages.

If it is accepted that moral discernment is something best carried out in communities, through social engagement, then drawing rigid boundaries around our ethical discourse, be they methodological, religious, ethnic or otherwise, is ultimately a self-negating and self-defeating strategy. Our ecclesial-ethical thinking is always in the world, often of the world and ought, always, to be *for* the world, as God has placed the creation in the stewardship of those created in God's likeness and called to present and eternal fellowship with God's being and with one another.

Let us see what theologically-informed ethics can offer to a broader debate about the developments in genetics, technology and the new and emergent bioethical and societal challenges posed by such. But let this not be an 'in-house' debate, conducted in a language or employing terminology only familiar to those insiders who perceive the world in the same way as those like ourselves. For one, it only leads to a very dull worldview and hence a dull existence within the safe haven of one's chosen community. But, second and much more importantly, the danger is that Christians thereby fail to fulfil their duty, because they deprive themselves of the opportunity to *inform* much wider moral challenges with the vast resources of theological wisdom and insight.

I have sought to help establish the case that some approaches to ethics result in those beyond the confines of the church refusing to listen to Christian perspectives; and so Christian moral voices have no impact, and hence contributions from Christians to the pressing moral debates are negated. Such seems contrary to the gospel – a going out into the world and cherishing all that is good and true. But, so too is the blind rejection of anything that is Christian, or indeed religious, being allowed to inform wider debates in the moral arena in pluralistic societies. It is hoped that the moral challenges raised by new developments in the genetic sciences will benefit from interdisciplinary conversation and discernment, and that it will become recognised that theologically-informed ethical voices have much to contribute to the ongoing debate.

R. JOHN ELFORD

Divine/Human Love and Creativity

The Christian faith is of central importance in the scientific writing of Gareth Jones. He thinks that it throws light on the nature of human responsibility in the face of contemporary technological challenges in the biological sciences. He writes: 'I am a scientist who is delving into theology and ethics; I am a neuroscientist who is dealing with genetics and developmental biology. And I am a Christian who sees virtue in scientific ventures.'[1] He invites comment upon this because he views ethics and theology as providing '… the ethos within which the science is undertaken'.[2] This chapter is one response to that invitation.

To understand that ethos we will need to explore some central themes in the New Testament and consider some of their implications for human conduct. Jesus' repeated injunction to his hearers that they should love one another is, of course, central to this ethos. 'I give you a new commandment, that you love one another. Just as I have loved you, you should also love one another.' (John 13:34) Understood in this way, human love becomes a reflection of the divine love in Jesus. For this reason, it is the fundamental motif of Christian ethics. The Greek word the gospels most commonly use for it is *agape*. This signifies the love of God to humankind, as distinct from brotherly love, *philos*, or erotic love, *eros*. However, it has importantly been pointed out that making too much of this distinction between *agape* and other forms of love can be misleading: firstly, because the usage did not strictly originate with Jesus and secondly, because there is much more to his teaching on love than is strictly associated with the word.[3] We

1   D. Gareth Jones, *Designers of the Future, Who Should Make the Decisions?* (Oxford: Monarch Books, 2005), p.9.
2   Ibid., p.203.
3   Victor Paul Furnish, *The Love Command in the New Testament* (London: SCM, 1973), p.222.

will see below that this second point is also true of the teaching of St Paul.

In the teaching of Jesus, love is importantly not an abstract concept. It is, rather, something that has to be instantiated in specific actions at particular times. Understanding this takes us to the heart of his method of teaching. He did not promulgate general theories and truths. What he did, rather, was to show his listeners how to go about realising God's love in the actual circumstances of their own lives. Moreover, he persistently told them that they had to work out how to do this for themselves. Whenever they asked him to do this for them, he refused. Nor should they, he frequently and emphatically added, look to authorities, such as religious ones, to do this for them either. Realising God's love required personal initiative and at times even controversial novelty.

The gospel writers all agree on the centrality of love in Jesus' teaching, but they each deal with it slightly differently. This is to be expected, of course, given that they wrote at different times for different purposes in ever changing circumstances. They all include the so-called 'double commandment', to love God and one's neighbour (Matthew 22:34–40, Mark 12:28–34, Luke 10:25–37) and stress that the former is not possible without the latter. The famous question put to Jesus by a young lawyer takes us right to the heart of the matter. 'Teacher, what shall I do to inherit eternal life?' (Luke 10:25) The lawyer answers this question with his own formulation of the Great Commandment. Jesus confirms the correctness of this and the matter could have rested there. But the lawyer, 'wanting to justify himself', went on to enquire: 'Who is my neighbour?' (v.29) The parable of the Good Samaritan was the famous reply. This is such a familiar story that we can easily miss its radical import. First, the exemplar of neighbourliness was not a priest or a Levite, but a Samaritan – effectively, that is, an outcast. In this radical way, Jesus showed how the love of God was part of the common lot of ordinary folk. It should, therefore, be sought amid their doings and not among those of the religious authorities. The break here with Jewish precedents could not have been clearer. In the story, the priest and the Levite have ostensibly good reasons for passing by on the other side of the road: the priest because he was bidden elsewhere and the Levite because he feared the ritual defilement that would be incurred if he touched what, by appearance, could have been a dead body. The Samaritan's response was prompted by ordinary human compassion. (v.34) What he did was an ordinary act of mercy. This is the everyday human stuff of neighbourliness and the key to the exercise of God's love. It is independent of racial considerations as well as of religious constraints. The traveller was presumably a Jew who was refused help by his co-religionists. None of them would have failed to noticed this on reading the parable. Here was a Samaritan, an outsider, portrayed as the exemplar of God's love by drawing on nothing other than his own humanity. The parable, therefore, stresses that when this happens all barriers of race, religion and conventional propriety are of no account. This simple and single act of mercy prompted by compassion exemplified God's love more clearly and radically than anything else. This archetypal story is of perennial fascination and relevance because it reminds its readers again and again of the style, simplicity, and profoundly innovative nature of Jesus' teaching. It shows that Jesus was not, in fact, a religious teacher as they were understood to be at the time. Both his teaching style and his message were more akin to those of the so-called Wisdom teachers in older Jewish tradition. This sort of teaching was once prominent in Jewish history. A great deal of the Old Testament is cast in its form. It was less prominent in Jewish circles by the time of Jesus. It is just possible that Jewish people who took offence at it were not as cognisant as they should have been of its precedent in their own traditions. The Wisdom teachers pointed to ordinary things and doings to illustrate their message. Above all, they valued accumulated human experience and considered it to be a profound source of divine wisdom.

The Gospels of both Luke and Matthew exhort their readers to 'love their enemies'. (Luke 6:27, Matthew 5:44) In this way they stress that there cannot ever be restrictions on who should be the recipients of God's love. It is not, therefore, something which can only be exercised among believers themselves. It has to be unlimited in its scope. An obvious implication of this is that there is nothing in human experience which can be impervious to God's love. All that experience, even when it is most ugly and repugnant to human sensibilities, is capable of redemption by God's love. This is to be achieved by ordinary human beings amid the everyday circumstances of their lives. It is eminently practical and down to earth. It invariably requires that something has to be done, it is also often spontaneous and is at its finest when carried out regardless of self-interest to the point of self-sacrifice. Matthew's Gospel is particularly illuminating at this point. For him, the love of God and of the neighbour is the same thing. It is also a practical thing; something which has to be attained through ordinary everyday acts of loving kindness. Those who act in this way may well be unaware of the profundity of their deeds. (Matthew 25:31–41) Theirs is a higher righteousness (5:20) that is achieved in loving actions towards those in need. Again and again Matthew stresses that loving acts towards the needy are the same thing as loving acts towards Christ. In this way, Matthew pushes the love ethic to its ultimate, and effectively secular, conclusion. To add to this that it is also the complete fulfilment of the law could not be more dramatic, particularly for a readership in what was undoubtedly the most Jewish of the early Christian communities.

The Gospel of John can be read as a gospel of love. Christians are to love one another as they have been loved. (13:34) This gospel, which is radically unlike the three others in so many ways, was probably intended to be read by Christians living in separate and perhaps even closed communities. For this reason, it has long been debated whether or not the love command is restricted to those communities, or whether it goes beyond them. Those who think the former see John's writing on love as a pale shadow of that in the other three gospels. The love of the like-minded is as nothing compared with the love of the outcast, the despised and even one's enemies, which, as we have seen, the other three gospel writers make so much of. Christian love is certainly weakened and even seriously compromised when its scope is restricted to Christian fellowship. Its greater work is unrestricted, as all the other gospel writers stress.

St Paul was to make much of all this in his teaching, though he does not quote the words of Jesus' teaching on love as such. Nor does he do so, of course, on any other topic. Paul's whole theology stems from the cross and the resurrection. It is systematic in the sense that its constituent parts fit together. It is also occasioned by the specific needs of the churches to which he addressed himself. He constantly writes about the tasks in hand and draws on his emerging thoughts as he does so. This makes him what would nowadays be called a pastoral theologian. It is always important to remember this when trying to understand what he wrote and thought. His great themes all hang together around the central one of 'justification by faith'. This alone was the all-sufficient means of salvation. (The Protestant Reformers were much later, of course, to make this central to their teaching.) Remember also that Paul was, with Barnabas, the architect of the mission to the Gentiles. After a momentous decision at the Council of Jerusalem in 49CE, the way was clear for the Christian gospel to be preached directly to Gentiles in a way which did not require them to be circumcised before accepting it. They could now be justified by faith alone without the law. By the cross and resurrection of Jesus all believers, in this way, were brought into a new life with him. This was the 'new being' or 'new creation' of which he made so much in his writing. It is sustained by the freely available love of God in Christ. (Galatians 6:15) Faith active in love is another central theme of his writing. At this point the systematic nature of his thinking becomes remarkably apparent. Paul sees the manifestation of love in the Christian life as the outpouring of the spirit. In all this, as in so much of Paul's life and work, we see Christian theology seminally in the making. So much so, in fact, that what he preached and taught, as well as the way in which he did so, is still clearly recognisable in Christian life and thought today. The letter to the Romans, c58CE, is his longest and theologically most comprehensive epistle. Whilst it was initially addressed to Christians in Rome in advance of his imminent visit to them, it has always been understood by the church to be of universal and timeless importance. The great Hymn to Love, to be found at 8:28–39, is one of the most resonant and well known pieces of writing in western literature. For Paul, love is what keeps believers in the embrace of God and what enables them to extend that to others. It is indestructible, and never more so than when Christians are suffering persecution, as Paul's readers in Rome were at the time he wrote.

Little wonder that love became the central motif in the life of the early Christian churches. All this is so familiar to us these many centuries later that we can easily overlook what a radical approach to morality this was at the time. Among other things it democratised

virtue, so to speak. It made virtue available to all, in particular the unlearned, and even the despised and the outcast. By the second century,
Christianity was noted for just this, the way it enabled ordinary people
to be virtuous. Gone were Jewish notions of virtue as being legal
observance. Love alone was the complete fulfilment of the law. It is
what creates the believer's freedom to live the life of faith in joyful
response to God's initial and enabling act of love in Christ. Brotherly
love and divine love are here at one with each other. It is what builds
up the life of the churches and what sets the agenda for their
relationship with the wider world. The resonance here with what
Mark, Matthew and Luke said about love could not be clearer. What
Paul did was to show how the love command could, through faith,
become the fulfilment of the law by enabling Gentiles to achieve
through it a New Righteousness. All this is nothing less than breath-
taking, and it shows, in brief, just how radical the early Christian
innovations in spirituality were. By these means ordinary human
beings could achieve a righteousness that went beyond anything that
had been envisaged before the Christian era. All this, of course, has
been familiar and essential to the life of the Christian churches ever
since. It has driven and still drives Christians to focus their spirituality
through hospitality, compassion and practical acts of pastoral care.
Christian religious observance is, therefore, essentially a practical
thing in the sense that no act of religious observance can ever be
complete without the inclusion of such acts of caring.

In the early centuries, as Christianity increasingly came into
contact with Greek thought, it was its understanding of love which set
it apart. Never before had there been anything quite like it. Here, as
we have seen, was a teaching on virtue which was freely available to
all, applicable to the ordinary circumstances of people's lives and
which facilitated a rejoicing that needed no other justification. Above
all, it required only baptism into the faith for its initiation. Gone were
all suppositions that love and virtue required lengthy instruction and
education. Believers were themselves to work out what the loving
thing was for them to do in the actual circumstances of their own
lives. Nothing could more sharply contrast with the Greek teaching on
virtue. For Plato, virtue could only be secured by the pursuit of knowledge, which is why he insisted that kings needed to be philosophers if

they were to reign with justice.[4] (What, of course, this view of virtue could not explain is why educated people are so very often the least virtuous.) On this view, virtue is hierarchical. It is dispensed from above and is essentially anti-democratic. This difference in understanding something as central to human life as the nature of virtue was part of the tension that arose between Christian and Greek cultures. This, however, did not precluded the two cultures from discovering other agreements, such as the understanding of 'being' which played a central part in the subsequent formulations of Christian orthodoxy. Such differing views over the nature of love had to be resolved if the two cultures were to cohere as they needed to do in the newly emerging civilised western world. Achieving just this was the great work of St Augustine. This work, like that of Paul before him, was to set the lasting standard of Christian orthodoxy.

Soon after the fall of Rome to the Goths in 410CE, Augustine began to write his magisterial *The City of God*. Its central argument showed why Christianity was not, as some claimed, responsible for the fall of Rome and also why it would not also fall. The book is constructed around the love motif. It differentiates human love, *eros*, from divine love, *agape*, and discusses their relationship. In this, the limitations of *eros* are overcome by *caritas* and taken up into *agape*. For Augustine, no human love is complete unless it is taken up into and includes the love of God. This does not mean that the love of earthly things is to be eschewed. On the contrary, they are to be loved because they are part of the greater love of God. Steeped as he was in classical as well as Christian learning, Augustine stressed that the classical virtues were incomplete unless they were redeemed by love. His understanding of love was nothing less that a synthesis of the New Testament and classical traditions. All the human virtues, he insisted, are as nothing unless they are infused with and transformed by the love of God.

Little wonder that, for the reasons we have briefly observed in the New Testament and early Christian history, love was and remains the central motif of Christian spirituality and virtue. In consequence, Christians often speak as though all we have to do, in one situation or

4   F. M. Cornford, *The Republic of Plato* (Oxford: Clarendon, 1961), pp.171ff.

another, is the loving thing; as though what that might be is always self-evident. What exactly that 'loving thing' might be, in this or that situation, is usually far from self-evident, however. The belief in self-evidence is a dangerous one. Whenever this predominates, mistaken certainty all too easily masquerades as virtue, and it does this never more so than when it is held collectively. All manner of rationalisations have been sought for this. One is the belief that some intuition will always lead the way to virtue. The danger here, of course, is that this can be a recipe for mass hysteria, as groups come to agree on love's requirement regardless of evidence to the contrary. Some of the worst atrocities in Christian history have been promulgated in this way. Even short of this, the belief that the loving thing to do is always self-evident has the effect of romanticising love and thereby divorcing it from the actual circumstances of any given situation. And of course, situations are often more complex than they might at first appear.

What precisely the loving thing to do might be in a particular situation is, therefore, invariably far from self-evident. For all the profundity of the Christian understanding of love, of itself it is so often incapable of yielding the required precision just when and where it is most needed. This is the simple reason why so many disputes can and do occur over the details of love's requirements. Love, alone, cannot always answer questions about what actually should, or should not, be done in specific situations. Rather, love leaves everything open. This is both its great strength and its weakness. Failure to recognise this is the source of so much misunderstanding in the name of love. This is no doubt why, in the teaching of Jesus, love's imperative is coupled with implied injunctions to 'think things out' as well. No amount of noble sentiment can obviate the need for this. This alone is good enough reason for Christians to engage in earnest debates about the requirements of virtue in given situations. Invariably, this entails a commitment to hard and sustained work alongside others who have the relevant factual information and who share goodwill. No intuited certainty can ever excuse those who want to do the loving thing from examining the facts. This is why the exercise of love requires intellect as well as passion, open-mindedness as well as certainty. It is also why those who seek to do the loving thing amid confusing circumstances should always welcome the assistance of any who can help dispel such confusion. This makes Christian morality hard-headed and realistic. It should always demand access to the very best of factual analyses. Only in this way can its options be identified and evaluated. All this, of course, gives the lie to the popular supposition that the Christian ethic is obscurantist and irrelevant to specific tasks in hand. Nothing, for the reasons we have seen, could be further from the truth. At their best, therefore, Christian preoccupations with the pursuit of virtue demand open hard-headedness. They also demand a degree of humility in the face of conflicting evidence. Only this can cut through the opinionating which so often obstructs any real progress with this issue or that. Whatever else God's wonderful world might be, it is certainly mysterious and full of surprises, for good as well as for evil. Seeking the former in all honesty and integrity is what the Christian pursuit of love requires.

But there is even more, much more, to the Christian understanding of love than this. It is as important to be clear about what love does do, as it is to be clear about what it cannot do. It does two things. First, it provides the inspiration for action. It prohibits us from standing by when others are in need. From a Christian point of view, doing something in these circumstances is a spiritual obligation. Second, love provides the means to sustain that action when the going gets tough. Here it even enjoins the undertaking of seemingly impossible tasks. These are the great works of love and it is always impressive and moving to see them in action. They are the stuff of human self-sacrifice in the service of others.

We have already begun to see why Christian love is not just esoteric. It is, rather, something which is engaged with the stuff of life itself at the very centre of human endeavour. It is something which always demands to be worked at. There are no short cuts to this. Some Christians, however, like to create the impression that there are; either by being romantic and unrealistic about love's requirements or by quoting words from scripture in ways which suggest that they constitute a sufficient answer in every circumstance and for all time. Moreover, they often further claim that if only we were to get back to scriptural basics in this way our problems would cease. Would that life were so simple – it is manifestly not! (We shall return to this point.) Jesus, as we have seen, repeatedly refused to give prescriptive advice on the issues of his own time. Furthermore, many of the dilemmas we face, particularly those arising from the new technologies, were not even prefigured in Jesus' time. Jesus' teaching is perennially relevant precisely because he did not engage in laying down time- and culture-bound prescriptions. What he did was something far more profound: he effectively told his enquirers to go away, love one another, think things out for themselves and throw themselves on the mercy of God. This latter point is important for the simple reason that human endeavour alone cannot secure virtue. It must always be directed towards seeking the sustaining grace of God.[5] When we set out to think things out for ourselves in this way we need all the help we can get. This is why the Christian understanding of virtue requires that the empirical facts of technology be taken seriously. This cannot be achieved by easy prejudgement. Rather, patience and humility are necessary in the face of ever emerging new information.

In practice, this means that Christian ethicists need to listen carefully to those with the expertise to explain the issues at stake. Only when they do this with integrity can they expect to be listened to by others. All this makes the Christian pursuit of virtue an interdisciplinary endeavour. This is extremely important, particularly in the modern world. It is now widely acknowledged that there are no single sources from which all-encompassing moral views can be derived. The moral life is too complex for that. Rather, what we have to do, when facing moral perplexity, is to be clear about where we start from and then be ready to draw on (many if necessary) other sources of inspiration. A good analogy here is that of a prism. What we see when we peer into a glass prism is that light is made up of a complex spectrum, of which we would otherwise be unable to separate the strands. Morality is much like this. Using this analogy of the prism to explain the anatomy of morality, one writer eloquently puts it this way:

> The prism … is … [but] an image, pointing to a complexity in our moral vision. The unseen white light can pass through the prism, but the complex of colours

5   R. John Elford, *The Ethics of Uncertainty* (Oxford: Oneworld, 2000), pp. 137–50.

remains; we may fasten selectively on one at any given time, yet we see it as but one colour in the spectrum. It does not eclipse the others, and if we are fortunate it can even enhance them.[6]

All this, in brief, is good enough reason for Christians to be engaged in earnest in debates such as those in the life sciences. Whilst they will have much to bring to the tables of discussion, they will also, equally, have much to learn about the mystery and infinite promise of God's mysterious, sometimes frightening, but beautiful world.

Understanding the relationship of Christian virtue to technology in these ways places it at the cutting edge of research and creativity. The human desire to be creative is predicated upon an awareness of a potential to change things, hopefully for the better. This creative potential is centred on the notion of problem solving. Things can be other than as they are. This is the very opposite of fatalism. It knows that things can be better. In other words, creative desire is ambitiously optimistic and focused. It is a dissatisfaction with the way things are, an impatience with convention. It is clearly an altruistic desire, particularly when directed to improving the lot of others. Gareth Jones's writing on the reproductive technologies is particularly strong on this point. He makes extensive use of case histories he has encountered as a clinician. This means that he is not discussing abstract principles; he is discussing very real human dilemmas. To want to do something for the better about them, when the technology exists for that purpose, is a natural human expression of concern for others. There can scarcely be any more noble human aspiration. Such a concern, however, cannot be exercised piecemeal, particularly in the reproductive technologies. There are issues at stake which affect the whole human race and even its indefinite future. (The prospective elimination of genetically transmitted disease is just one such.)

The Christian understanding of creativity derives from a belief in the sovereignty of God. To be sovereign, God has to be the Lord of Creation. This is a familiar theme throughout the Old Testament, particularly in the Psalms, which are redolent with references to the wonder and amazement of creation. The 'created order' is the phrase

6   Dorothy Emmet, *The Moral Prism* (London: Macmillan, 1979), p.158.

most often used in the Christian tradition to refer to this. It draws attention not only to the fact that its initial existence was at the behest of God, but also to the claim that its continued existence is also at God's behest. It is, of course, self-evident that the created order is far from perfect. Long gone are the days when the romantic imagination could gloss over this. Tennyson's great phrase from the poem *In Memoriam* about nature being 'red in tooth and claw' is now the widely accepted view. We cannot possibly know why God chose, as God must have done, to create the world in this way. To believe in God is to believe that God just did. The world is imperfect. So too are human beings. However, for all their flaws and limitations, human beings know that they possess very considerable creative powers, which go beyond their ability to reproduce themselves. They know, too, that they have some sort of moral obligation to exercise these powers.

The Judaeo-Christian tradition is particularly good at articulating all this. Christians understand their obligation to be creative as something more than a moral obligation; it is, rather, a divine imperative. Something, that is, which has to be done to honour and fulfil the divine/human relationship. This is why creative impassivity is not an option for Christian believers. Some of them, with others, can often be heard to say that nature should be left as it is, but this is not an option, for the reasons explained above. Given that the created order is as it is, the very best has to be made of it. Leaving nature to take its own course is not even a realistic option. Indeed, if this had ever been an option, human history would have ceased long ago. Humankind's survival is a testimony to human inventiveness (as, similarly, is the ever increasing longevity of individual human beings). The created order is full of naturally successful predators upon humans, such as viruses. These would reign supreme were it not for human ingenuity in creating the conditions to check them. People who want nature to be left to its own devices are simply drawing some arbitrary line between what should be left alone and what should not be. They scarce add anything to the debate, beyond reminding us that nature should be reverenced; an important point that was never at issue in this debate anyway. Whatever other merits and de-merits the Christian understanding of human life and the created order might possess, and there are many, this point about the necessity of intervention and its links to the human urge to be creative is particularly illuminating at this juncture. The human capacity for creativity is, therefore, helpfully understood as something God-given.

Gareth Jones's scientific research is at the cutting edge of his subject. He seeks, always, to discover new ways of alleviating human disease, handicap and distress. The biological technologies in which he works are yielding ever more new possibilities for achieving these ends. This is the sense in which they are immensely creative. As we have seen, Christian thought and practice profoundly embraces the notion of creativity. For this reason it is a significant part of the Christian ethos to which Jones, as a scientist, turns for inspiration. The Christian doctrine of creation sets out to achieve nothing less than an explanation of why things exist and to what purpose they do so: it is about much more than whether or not the world was created in six days, or whether the events recorded in the first two chapters of Genesis can be verified or disproved empirically. Thus, Christians claim not just to know why things exist, but also to know what to do about this awesome and otherwise inexplicable fact of existence. This is a doctrine is of immense Christian significance, going far beyond the parameters within which it is usually confined. For our purpose, its most relevant aspect is the belief that human beings were created in the divine image. This alone sets the scene for understanding what responsibilities human beings have towards the created order.

Because human beings are understood to be created in the divine image, it means that, in some sense, they are to share with God the responsibility for the wellbeing of creation. 'So God created man in his own image, in the image of God he created him, male and female he created them.' (Genesis 1:27) This is followed in the text by the information that Adam then created sons, obviously in his own image. (Genesis 4:1ff) The implication of this for the biblical understanding of human nature is clear. All subsequent human beings are likewise created in the divine image. It is, of course, totally inappropriate and misleading to ask only whether all this is historically true. The more profound question is what does it all mean? It means nothing less than the fact that human beings have a very special role to play as they live out their short lives in the infinitely greater purpose of the created order. This presents them with both immense privileges and awesome responsibilities.

The Jewish understanding that humankind was created in the divine image (Genesis 1:27) is the reason for its prohibition of both divine and human images. (Exodus 20:4ff) The presence of God in worship is, rather, shown by the use of candles and the Ark of the Covenant. For Jews, God is known through his actions in history and through his continuing providence for them as his chosen people. Precisely what 'image' means in this context is, of course, debatable. It is generally agreed however that is refers to every aspect of being human. This is the reason why humankind is able to exercise divine capacities, particularly in relation to the created order towards which we have a special responsibility. Humankind exercises God's claim to dominion over the earth. The main emphasis here is on the fact that, although human beings are like God in every respect, they are like God essentially in what they do. An expression of the marvel of this is found in Psalm 8:4–6:

> ... what is man that thou art mindful of him, and the son of man that thou dost care for him? Yet thou hast made him a little less than God, and dost crown him with glory and honour. Thou hast given him dominion over the works of thy hands; thou hast put all things under his feet.

Psalm 8 begins and ends with praise for the majesty of God, and this central motif celebrates humankind's unique responsibilities in this regard. This makes humankind vulnerable, fragile and ever dependent on God's sustaining grace. In this way, human dignity is seen to be of divine origin. Praising this is a natural and central reaction in Jewish spirituality. None of this was to be represented pictorially, it was to be celebrated in the knowledge that human and divine actions were, for all humankind's frailty, interlinked. Throughout Jewish anthropology the fact that humankind has divine-like responsibilities is accepted and celebrated. One could scarcely find, or even imagine, a higher view of human nature than this.

Christian anthropology inherited all this. It too avoided repre-sentations of the divine image. These did not begin to appear until the second century in catacomb decoration, and even then their propriety was questioned. The emphasis, rather, was on what human beings had to do in response to God's saving action in Christ. As we have already seen, love was the central key to understanding how they should relate to God and to one another. The reason why the New Testament does not take up reflection on the import of this for responsibilities towards the created order is simply, of course, because none of its writers, with the possible exception of the writer of Luke/Acts, expected the created order to last – the parousia, the return of the Lord in glory, was thought to be imminent. As it was delayed further and further, we can see how, in fact, they were forced to pay more and more attention to earthly responsibilities and conduct. But none of this emerging reflection ever equalled the older Jewish extended understanding of humankind's responsibilities towards creation. In Colossians 1:15 Christ is described as being the image of the invisible God. The use of image here does not just mean a copy or representation. It is meant, rather, to show that Christ is a living likeness of the invisible God. For this reason, in his person divine and human attributes, such as love, were at one. The knowledge of Christ as the Son of God was a knowledge of God. Responding to this in love was a response to the divine initiative in Christ. For St Paul, the divine image in humankind is marred by sin but restored through obedience to Christ. (Romans 8:29) By this means, all things are to work together for the good. To behold the glory of God in Christ is at the same time to participate in it. 'And we all, with unveiled face, beholding the glory of the Lord, are being changed into his likeness, from one degree of glory into another; for this comes from the Lord who is the spirit.' (2 Corinthians 3:18) For Paul, fellowship with Christ is the means whereby the restoration of the divine likeness in humankind is achieved. He did not let this rest at the point of spiritual speculation. Throughout his writings he stressed repeatedly that this above all had consequences for human conduct. Because human beings living in Christ were who they were, they had a special relationship to and responsibility for one another. Christian fellowship was the living reality of the redeemed human life in Christ. Paul stresses again and again the responsibility which Christians have to bear one another's burdens. (Galatians 6:2) This is the foundation of the central pastoral element in Christian spirituality. Caring for others is not, therefore, a consequence of

Christian spirituality, it is of its very essence. This is because all human beings are created in the image of God. To care for them is therefore to strive for the restoration of that image, however blurred by circumstance it might have become. This is why, in his writings, Paul is never content simply to proclaim the gospel, important to him thought that clearly was. He invariably goes on to help his readers to understand what its implications are for their lives in their own circumstances and times. The goal of all this was the attainment of righteousness, a being put right with God. This was not initially an ethical righteousness, though it had ethical implications. It was first and foremost a spiritual condition, enabling new life in Christ and a new being in the life of the believer. Again and again, Paul wrote to Christian communities who were perplexed by what their new life in Christ demanded of them. To this end he was always ready to explore and develop his theology and to apply it to the ever changing circumstances of the lives of those for whom he cared. In this way he exemplified and established the central place of the pastoral in Christian life and thought. For him, what Christians believed and what they did were two sides of a coin. Neither could exist without the other. As we have seen, he showed a remarkable awareness of how changing circumstances created ever new challenges in the Christian life. Tackling these, for him, was of the essence of Christian spirituality. He never suggests that they could be settled once and for all. What he shows throughout his writing is that they have to be worked at constantly. He calls for a sort of pastoral vigilance at the very heart of Christian spirituality.

These seemingly profound insights create, however, a number of problems. Human beings are not God. For them to think otherwise is for them to commit the sin of spiritual pride. They are differentiated from God by some stark contrasts. Unlike God, they were created and, therefore, are dependent creatures. Furthermore, they are manifestly sinful, of limited foresight and circumscribed ability. Even at its very best, therefore, human creativity can only be a reflection of its divine provenance. The reason for this is a simple one. Everything human beings do and create reflects their own nature, including its imperfections. This means, of course, that they cannot create something which is flawless. They cannot eliminate the dark side from their own natures, nor from its reflection in their creations. For this reason, the ambivalence of good and evil is as manifest in the objects of human creation as it is in human nature itself. This is what makes the striving for perfection in human creativity such an elusive goal. This striving is one of the deep springs of creativity, but the perfect '*x*' can never be created. This does not mean that the striving will ever cease. To the contrary, it is the main reason for its perennial quest. This is the proverbial 'holy grail' of the poetic imagination, the 'stone' of the philosophical mind. All this is comparatively straightforward in, for example, the performing and visual arts. Failures here are harmless, though they might be embarrassing and expensive. They simply fall by the wayside of critical derision and may or may not ever be resurrected. Elsewhere, however, such failures are not harmless when they affect the human condition adversely. They soon become notorious and invariably cause an adverse reaction, which generates repugnance towards their perpetrators and their methods.

In the foregoing we have considered a little of what it means to see Christian love and its requirements at the heart of the Christian life. We have also seen what a radical novelty this was in the early centuries of the Christian church. Above everything else, it was, and still is, a dynamic. It has proved itself capable of adapting to new situations and rising to new challenges. This is important. Its requirements are never settled once and for all, nor are they capable of definitive formulations that hold good for all time and in all circumstances. The requirements of love are much more mercurial. All this tells us something important about the way in which Christians should understand the Bible and subsequent Christian tradition.

There is of course a widespread Christian view that the Bible is the final authority in all things and that it contains everything needed for life guidance and eternal salvation. On this view, all one has to do in a specific situation is to look up the relevant passages and carry out what they require. The word most commonly used to describe this view is 'fundamentalism'. Whilst this comes in many forms, they are all predicated on the belief in an all-sufficient scripture. Everything we need for our salvation is therein, and hence we need look nowhere else for it. Invariably, those who hold such views do so inflexibly and even pedantically. They are also, for the most part, anti-scientific, and the controversies they engender are well known and seemingly perennial. They need not detain us here. What we do, however, need to look into are the main reasons why such an approach to the Bible is unacceptable.

Firstly, the Bible is not a homogenous whole. Its writings span some two millennia. They differ greatly in their motivation, literary style, and historical contexts. Individual writers, moreover, were not interested in or even always cognisant of the works of other biblical writers. They focused, rather, on their own purpose for writing in and for their own life and times. When they were writing, they would have been unaware that their work would eventually be assembled with that of other writers, as it now is. 'Scripture' was a later notion imposed upon the assemblage of writing when it was given canonical status. That is an interesting story in its own right, but one which cannot be allowed to engage us further here. All we need to note are the reasons for not accepting the view that the Bible is made up of homogenous writings that are coherent and consistent on everything they discuss. Long gone are the days when writers wrote about the biblical view of this or that as though it were homogenous. There are, of course, important and consistent themes in the Bible about God's saving grace and actions. These, however, are the background, important though that is, to the outworking of their import in the lives of the faithful here and now. What, in fact, we get to see, when we read and study the Bible carefully, is the life of faith in its formation in this situation or that, at one or other particular time. The biblical writers were all doing their best, in their own circumstances, for those for whom they wrote.

They could not have been expected to do more than this. The marvel is that they invariably did it so well that their writings have been valued and preserved as they have been. All this can be countered, of course, by the retort that they were divinely inspired. That can mean several things. If it means that they were inspired to do their very best, that is acceptable. If, however, it is taken to mean that they were inspired to reveal all truth for all time in complete agreement with one another, that is less so. They are, in fact, often in disagreement. Their views, moreover, can be seen to change and develop. This is nowhere clearer than it is in the New Testament. As the imminent return of the Lord in glory was delayed, then so they had to change their views to adapt to ongoing and ever demanding circumstances. What we therefore discover in the Bible is that the faith of its writers was always 'in the making'. None of them did it once and for all and for everybody. They all wrote as they did because they had something new and important to say which had not been previously said in the situation in which they found themselves. We do not actually know why, for example, the gospels were written at all. It is clear, however, that they were occasioned in the sense that we have just described. Indeed, when subsequent writers followed Mark, the earliest of the gospels, they respected what he had written, but felt free to change and rearrange it in their own narratives. St Paul, as we have seen, was another exemplar, showing how the faith could be re-explored and understood in one situation or another.

What all this shows is that the biblical faith has ever been in the making. It has never at any one point been made in a way that can last for ever, in all circumstances. As these change, the job has to be re-visited. The biblical writers are an inspiration to us because they show us how to do this. They are an example and guide. Just are they were constrained to do things differently and more appropriately than their predecessors, then so should we be. The point is that the biblical faith needs just as much making in our own life and times as it did in theirs. We emulate them, therefore, not by slavishly copying them but by using them as our inspiration to achieve in our own times what they achieved in theirs. Like them, we will not always get everything right. Others will have to come after us as the making of the biblical faith goes on, as it will ever need to do this side of the Kingdom of God. All this is sufficient reason to see why the Bible is as important as it is in the making of that faith. Its creative dynamic must be ours as we seek to emulate its example.

In the Introduction to this book, Gareth Jones has drawn attention to the present dramatic speed of inexorable technological innovation in the medical (as well as other) sciences. This is now a fact of life, and we simply have to cope with it – it is not going to go away. We have to prepare ourselves for things to get yet more challenging as new technologies come to the fore. Lead-times for developments are ever shortening. For this reason we can confidently expect that in a very short time into the unseen future we will have to be coping with technological innovations in the medical, and other, sciences which are as yet unheard of. Unless we devise effective ways of managing these technologies, they will become a burden rather than a benefit to human welfare. This is why so much attention is paid to this issue throughout this volume.

In this chapter we have seen that the Christian faith is appropriate in this context not because it can deliver eternal and unchanging certainties in matters of fine detail; it is relevant precisely because it does not do this and because it enables us to cope with uncertainty and novelty. It does this principally in two ways. It enables us on the one hand to deal with the ambiguity we so often find when we read the Bible and, on the other, to deal also with the uncertainty we face when we have to commit to courses of action. The Christian moral tradition, understood in this way, is lively, open, challenging and ever relevant to changing circumstances. It enables those who earnestly seek to do the right thing in changing and challenging circumstances to search for and apply solutions which, provisional though they might often be, nevertheless enable us to exercise our God-given gift of creativity in the service of others. This can only be done prayerfully and humbly in the hope that, at their best, our doings will be redeemed by God's grace. When we catch glimpses of this happening, we see how our often confusing world is redeemed, little by little, and enabled to reveal the greater purposes of the love that God has for all God's creatures. As we seek to do the right things in these and other circumstances we cannot realistically ever hope for more than this. It is, however, more than we need to be going on with, and this is why medicine and faith draw such insight from each other in partnership.

Adam Hood

A Personalist Approach to Bioethics

This chapter looks at the contribution of the Scottish theologian John Oman[1] to bioethical discussions. This is not a topic that has been dealt with before, since there has been relatively little published on Oman, and what has been produced has tended to have a doctrinal rather than an ethical focus.[2] Nevertheless, given that Oman was pre-eminently concerned with theological anthropology, a relevance to bioethics may be assumed. Moreover, a discussion of Oman allows for some reflection on what might be expected of any theology in relation to bioethical discourse.

The thesis has three aspects. Firstly, that Oman's emphasis on autonomy as *the* human good helps us to clarify one important value that will play a part in bioethical discourse. There are however limits to the usefulness of this way of viewing the *summum bonum*, which reflects the fact that there is no one way of encompassing harmoniously the variety of legitimate ethical ends that enter into such debates. It is assumed, following Berlin, that legitimate ethical ends are sometimes logically incommensurable.[3] Secondly, Oman's fluid understanding of the concept of the 'natural', it is held, provides a positive framework within which to discuss developments in the biosciences. Thirdly, his understanding of 'sincerity' encourages sensitivity to the actualities of scientific progress and the multiplicity of concerns that play a role in bioethical decision making.

---

1 John Oman (1860–1939), Presbyterian minister and principal of Westminster College, Cambridge, from 1922 to 1935.
2 See, for instance, Stephen B. Bevans, *John Oman and His Doctrine of God* (Cambridge: CUP, 1992); and Adam Hood, *Baillie, Oman and Macmurray* (Aldershot: Ashgate, 2003).
3 Bernard Williams, 'Introduction' to Isaiah Berlin, *Concepts and Categories: Philosophical Essays*, ed. Henry Hardy (Oxford: OUP, 1980), pp.xi–xviii, p.xvi.

There are reports from bioscientists of the limited value of much bioethical reflection, especially that coming out of the theological world. The reasons for this will be varied, but of significance, in the view of Gareth Jones, is the tendency of theological opinion to be 'reactionary, responding to extreme scenarios'.[4] Perhaps one explanation is the wide influence, in the theological world, of an approach to ethics typified by the work of Stanley Hauerwas.[5] Hauerwas argues that, from a Christian point of view, ethics is defined by the gospel of Jesus Christ and addresses, rather than converses with, other perspectives. In principle this view rules out the possibility of progress in moral insight, beyond, that is, a growing understanding of what is thought to be implicit in Christ, the biblical text and the Christian tradition. There is a connection between such a view and a reactionary approach to bioscience. If one has a relatively fixed view of ethical norms and is disquieted about the discoveries of secular people and disciplines, then one will tend to be suspicious of developments in bioscience, especially if these seem to challenge or require modifications in established Christian positions. Yet it does seem incredible to deny that human beings have, historically, grown in their understanding of the world, including of themselves, and that our apprehension of the Christian gospel will be modified thereby. Indeed the church has, as a matter of course, modified her faith in response to intellectual and social discoveries. The church's accommodation to evolutionary theory is a case in point. The Christian tradition has found it expedient to exist in a creative dialogue with modernity. Pope Benedict comments: 'All that is great in modernity must be acknowledged unreservedly.'[6] Meanwhile, Barbour hints at the modest role that faith may play in relation to modern knowledge:

---

4   D. Gareth Jones, 'Enhancement: Is Baseless Speculation Misleading Theologians and Bioethicists?', this volume, p.126.
5   See R. John Elford, *The Ethics of Uncertainty* (Oxford: Oneworld, 2000), pp. 54–57.
6   Quoted in *The Tablet*, 23 Sept 2006, p.12.

We cannot expect to find in the Bible any easy answers to complex issues today, but we can try to identify in it some of the values that can guide us in our choices.[7]

Theology, then, exists as a dialogue partner with science. In this dialogue there is sense in making use of the whole available repertoire of theological resource. It is in this regard that my soundings in the work of John Oman may have value.

An assumption in what follows has to do with the nature of the contribution that theology can make to ethical discussions. Barbour helpfully suggests that there have been three broad approaches to ethics within the Christian community, which focus, respectively, on 'choice of the good, obedience to the right, and search for the fitting response'.[8] My own view is that we do not have to choose amongst these three approaches, since each touches on a dimension of the moral circumstances that people wrestle with. The role of theological ethics, as understood here, is to clarify important dimensions of actual ethical situations that we otherwise might miss, and it does this through drawing on a varied selection of theoretical insights. That is, theology's role is not to define the good, nor to tell us what we must do, nor even to make judgements on the basis of metaphysics, but to help sharpen our awareness of the ethical dimensions of discussions such as those surrounding the clinical technique known as pre-implantation genetic diagnosis. From this perspective, theology does not define the ethical terrain, nor does it offer ready-made solutions to ethical dilemmas, but it may contribute, in its own distinctive way, some tools that will assist in the ethical discussions that are perennial to any community. I am here, in a manner, following David Hume in arguing that theological ethics has an empirical focus. It may well be that an approach that defines a *summum bonum*, a set of duties or a collection of appropriate responses in abstraction 'may be more perfect in itself, but [it] suits less the imperfection of human nature'.[9]

---

7   Ian Barbour, *Ethics in an Age of Technology* (London: SCM, 1992), p.45.
8   Ibid., p.42.
9   David Hume, *Enquiries Concerning the Human Understanding and Concerning the Principles of Morals*, 2nd edn (London: OUP, 1902), p.174.

It is from this point of view that I will argue that John Oman has a useful contribution to make to bioethical discourse.

I shall find it useful, in order to bring out the points I wish to make, to discuss Oman in relation to a particular issue in bioethics. For the purposes of this chapter, I choose to discuss pre-implantation genetic diagnosis, which has been a matter of some controversy in recent times. Gareth Jones summarises this technique and the issues surrounding it in the following way:

> PGD is a procedure devised to test early human embryos for serious inherited genetic conditions. Only embryos that are free from the condition are transferred to a woman, in the expectation that a normal pregnancy will result. Inevitably, this involves selecting embryos: selecting those that are not genetic carriers of the disease trait, and discarding those that have the gene responsible for the disease. Herein lies the perceived problem: *selection*. Some embryos are chosen for further development; others are not. Some will be given the chance of becoming a new human being; others will be denied that chance.[10]

PGD is a technique used in tandem with IVF for beneficial therapeutic purposes. It allows certain genetic conditions, such as Huntington's disease, to be tackled effectively. Such uses will be, for many people, unexceptionable from an ethical perspective. For others, any technique that involves selection of some embryos and the discarding of others is suspect. Suspicion is heightened by the fear that selection might, in principle, be used for reasons other than those of viability or the avoidance of the birth of a person suffering or prospectively suffering from a genetically determined condition. Some people fear the use of PGD to determine the sex of a baby or, more fantastical, to design a baby with certain desirable biological characteristics (looks, intelligence, strength and so forth); this, for them, is the probable outcome of selection. Selection leads, in this view, to the commodification of life. Moreover, there are also fears about the practical implications of the way of thinking that informs PGD for those who suffer from genetic disorders. How will their lives be valued in a world where medicine aims to prevent the birth of any others of their kind?

10   D. Gareth Jones, 'Is PGD a Form of Eugenics?', this volume, pp.143–44.

Autonomy as *the* Human Good

The various trajectories of Oman's work can be seen as converging on the question of what it is to live a good human life, or to exhibit 'moral personality'.[11] The salience of this question for Oman is illustrated in his view of Christ's significance. Oman's Christology focuses on Jesus' example of honest and courageous living. It is not what he did for us, nor what he taught, but his exemplary mode of life that is significant. Oman's analysis of moral personality lays stress on at least three dimensions. For him the moral personality lives autonomously, responsibly and is sustained by personal relationships.

Oman's view of autonomy suggests that it includes three moments. Firstly, to be autonomous is to exhibit self-consciousness.

> When we say the moral person lives in the world of his own self-consciousness, more is meant than that every person is conscious of self, or even that the self is the centre of all experience. It means that the world I deal with is all of it my world, towards all of which I can be active, if only by way of approval or disapproval.[12]

Human beings, on this view, form intentions and act on the basis of their personal interpretation of their environment. There are, of course, a number of facets that contribute to the 'meaning' that is given to the world. Material and ideal interests, events and emotions will all go to shape how a person reads their material and human environment. Moreover, self-consciousness is a concept which is both descriptive and prescriptive. All people, for Oman, live out of an interpretation of their environment. Few, however, pursue an autonomous interpretation of the world; many, if not most, are the 'hollow men' of T. S. Eliot's imagination.

Secondly, autonomy involves self-direction. Self-direction is the capacity that human beings have to legislate for themselves, that is, to form their own intentions. Oman's use of the figure of 'legislation' in

---

11   Oman distinguishes between ethical and moral, the latter being a more encompassing term than the former, which refers to necessary rules of conduct.

12   John Oman, *Grace and Personality*, 4th edn (Cambridge: CUP, 1931), p.54.

this regard is an apt one, since self-direction involves the capacity to judge between actions and determine which to choose.[13] The opposite of self-direction, heteronomy – 'legislation for us by others' – is, for Oman, the essence of sin.

In the light of his argument that human beings are best self-directed, Oman views conscience as the given state of a person's moral insight at any particular time.[14] It is not a given and fixed set of intuitions or rules. Moreover the conscience can be educated but not instructed. This paradoxical statement is an attempt to emphasise that whilst a person will necessarily learn from life and from others, yet there ought to be something essentially autonomous about the way in which a person interprets their world and the intentions that they form. Each person must come to their own considered view; even the divine will cannot short-circuit this moral necessity.[15]

Oman tries to underpin his argument against heteronomy by pointing to some of the drawbacks of allowing others to shape our conscience.[16] Allowing the views or determinations of others to shape our conscience will narrow the scope of our awareness of our environment. We will be ignorant of the new challenges and insights that changing circumstances are throwing up, since our ways of thinking, feeling and acting are being set for us by others and not by our interaction with the environment. Indeed, heteronomy in its extreme form involves the individual thinking and acting in such a way as to please other people. Oman's perspective is, in contrast, consistent with that of Walt Whitman, who writes:

> Not I, nor any one else can travel that road for you,
> You must travel it for yourself...
> You are also asking me questions and I hear you,
> I answer that I cannot answer, you must find out for yourself.[17]

---

13   Oman, *Grace and Personality*, p.51.
14   It is important to note that by conscience or moral awareness Oman has in mind the general relation that people have to issues of truth, beauty and goodness.
15   John Oman, *The Natural and the Supernatural* (Cambridge: CUP, 1931), p.316.
16   Oman, *Grace and Personality*, p.45.
17   Walt Whitman, 'Song of Myself', in *Complete Poetry and Prose*, ed. James E. Miller (Boston: Houghton Mifflin, 1959), p.64.

Thirdly, autonomy involves self-determination – the capacity to act in terms of the self's intentions. Oman regards the awareness that is associated with self-determination as 'our most direct conscious experience' and indeed the basis of self-consciousness.[18] That is, the self becomes aware of itself through its actions, which mark it out as distinct from the environment. It follows that self-identity is the memory of the self's successive doings in the world. Oman stresses, in this regard, that the self's being is constituted by the will, by the capacity for self-determination.

Autonomy, as Oman describes it, is a goal greatly valued in societies such as ours. It is cherished as an expression of individuality, but also as a means to gaining fresh insight and understanding as is generated in an 'open society'. Moreover Oman provides a theological context for autonomy when he argues that, ontologically speaking, the possibility of human autonomy arises from God's will that the world should be a place where autonomy is possible. The world, for Oman, is a personal world because it allows, supports and responds to human autonomy. All this suggests that autonomy is a value that will play a role in bioethical discussions. To take PGD as an example, it can be argued that one legitimate impetus behind the development of this technology is the desire to enhance the autonomy of those who are born, and it is difficult to deny that the eradication of genetic disorders is a positive contribution to this worthy end.

On the other hand, autonomy cannot be the only or overriding value in the discussion of PGD. Taken to its logical conclusion, it might be possible to argue that embryo selection on the grounds of gender or an admired human characteristic could be justified in order to achieve the maximum autonomy of a child. In some societies, for instance, being a male might be counted as a necessary condition for self-determination. That most people will feel such developments are morally suspect shows that autonomy cannot be the only value that plays a role in such discussions. The intuition that embryos, including those that are discarded in clinical procedures, have an intrinsic dignity cannot arise from an emphasis on autonomy. Since an embryo is clearly not in the position of an autonomous person, at best it could

18   Oman, *Grace and Personality*, p.45.

only be considered to have potentiality; any dignity that it possesses cannot be understood as arising from the expression of autonomy. Moreover, were autonomy to be considered the sole expression of human being, it would be impossible to argue for the full humanity of those suffering from mental or physical limitations that preclude them from being fully or even partially self-determined. I am thinking here, for instance, of those who suffer from progressed senile dementia or who are born with severe learning difficulties. And yet the fact that we intuitively do ascribe dignity and value to such people, and to the human embryo, shows that there is a plurality of considerations that we take into account in our discussions.

Oman's Concept of the Natural

A basic difference in theological outlooks is that between those who think of the discipline as an exploration of that which has been given in Christ once and for all, and those who understand matters in more fluid ways. I tend towards the latter, seeing theology as one of the reflective exercises by which human beings aim to construct and reconstruct images of themselves in relationship with other human beings and with the created world in general, in part as a response to new understandings in the sciences. In this sense theology stands alongside and shares much with other imaginative and creative cultural forms such as literature, the arts, philosophy and political economics. Its concern is with the ways that human beings interpret and respond to their environment. In this sense it is distinguished from the natural sciences, which are properly concerned with understanding the fundamental physical structures of the universe. On the other hand, the motivation behind and legitimacy of the natural sciences is dependent, to some extent, on how human beings interpret them-selves; and this is certainly the case when it comes to biotechnologies. My argument is that Oman's idea of the 'natural' provides a theo-logical framework that encourages bioscientific work and enables a positive if not uncritical evaluation of progress in this area. It leans in the direction of understanding nature (and the divine will) as, in the words of Bookchin:

> An aeons long process of ever-greater differentiation: from the primal energy pulse that supposedly gave rise to the 'Big Bang', to the emergence of subatomic particles and the forces that bind the universe, to the complex elements that are known to us in the periodic table, to the appearance of all the celestial bodies of which we have knowledge, to the combinations of elements into molecules, amino acids, proteins and so forth – up to or until the emergence of organic and sentient beings on our planet ... in short ... a cumulative evolutionary process from the inanimate to the animate and ultimately the social.[19]

There are two aspects of Oman's thought that I want to stress here. First, for him, our perceptions, as a human race, of ourselves and the world are continually being revised and this constant revolution is propelled by the incursion of the divine into human experience. Second, the 'natural' has no inherent stability, for the evolution of the world is ongoing through human agency.

Autonomy, for Oman, has a two-sided relationship to knowledge. It is the precondition of a growth in knowledge, since the freedom to ask questions and pursue novel answers is fundamental to creative innovation. On the other hand, it is the human capacity to look beyond the given to what might be, which makes autonomous living possible. It is the human capacity to imagine new ways of understanding and acting that is the sufficient condition of autonomy. Psychologically this capacity for 'fresh expressions' arises from a feeling of awe in response to the natural world, which in its turn generates curiosity, the desire for understanding. From a theological perspective Oman understands this feeling of awe as the intuition of the good, the true and the beautiful; that is, the divine.

Oman is working here with a dialectic of the natural and the supernatural. The natural is the given state of the world at any one time, which he sees as the product both of physical and spiritual evolution.[20] The supernatural is that in human experience that draws

19 Murray Bookchin, *The Ecology of Freedom: The Emergence and Dissolution of Hierarchy* (Oakland and Edinburgh: AK Press, 2005), p.22.
20 John Oman, *Vision and Authority*, 2nd edn (London: Hodder, 1928), chapter 1.

us towards truth, goodness and beauty, and that enables autonomous forms of thinking, feeling and acting. It is the divine or supernatural which calls us continually to new ways of understanding the meaning of things. Oman's view is that the full meaning of life will only become clear in the eschaton. This is to say that current understandings are always partial, provisional and anticipatory of further insight and knowledge. From an epistemological point of view, that which is, the natural, is only the current state of knowledge and it is inherently unstable. Through the autonomous exercise of the imagination, humans are constantly beckoned beyond. This explains why Oman views heteronomy as the epitomy of 'sin'. It is not only the infringement of moral personality, it also prevents fresh insight into the divine will.

The idea that the reality of the environment is progressively being disclosed through the exercise of human autonomy places a premium on the new and innovative in human life. This perspective encourages a positive and welcoming attitude towards the endeavours of the human spirit, one that expects to find in these much that is enlarging. This is a perspective that would encourage hopefulness towards bioscientific developments. It stresses the potential for good in humankind, which is itself a reflection of the divine activity within human experience. It does not ignore sin, but sees it as arising out of the refusal to embrace the unfolding future. Closure of the mind, as a protective strategy, is an enduring human problem. It is the attempt to retreat behind walls of certainty, whether in ethics, doctrine or ecclesiology. Such retreat arises, in Oman's view, from the perennial fear of the future and of change.

Oman's view that the divine will is known through intellectual and emotional openness has important implications for bioethical debate. Jones's observation of the theological tendency towards drawing conclusions from extreme scenarios might suggest that discussion has been inhibited by negative prejudice which precludes careful scrutiny of the actual issues. In this way a negative and simplistic response to 'selection', 'commodification' and 'enhancement' leads almost automatically to the search for extreme scenarios that bear out prejudices. What is needed is a more impartial consideration of 'selection' and other controversial subjects. My view is that Oman's reflections on the coincidence of intellectual curiosity and the divine will provides the context in which such investigations can go on; whilst others theologies, in practice, close down the discussions before they have a proper chance to begin. In his recent Miliband Lecture, Stephen Lukes has pointed out that the term commodification, which some take as an expression of the inherently corrosive nature of the marketisation of some goods and services, such as health, is more ambiguous than sometimes appears. Lukes argues, persuasively, that the negative connotation of 'commodification' arises from assumptions that are sometimes paternalistic and often simplistic. He calls for an honest appreciation of the way in which the impersonal and quantifiable exist habitually in an uneasy but sustainable relationship with the personal, the altruistic, and the striving after values that are 'higher, personal and shared'.[21]

Analogously it might be argued that there is a need for greater theological scrutiny of key concepts in the discussion of PGD and other bioscientific developments. The assumption, in relation to PGD, that 'selection', 'commodification' and 'enhancement' are *de facto* illegitimate from a Christian point of view needs proper scrutiny, bearing in mind the actualities of scientific development and human experience.

Oman holds that the concept of the 'natural' denotes no more than the current stage of physical and social evolution. In this sense the 'natural' does not suggest stasis so much as anticipate further evolution. Oman's conception of the personal way in which God relates to humankind suggests that 'evolution' is brought about through the human quest for, and commitment to live in terms of, new insight. This way, there is a progressive disclosure of the supernatural in the visible world. God's will and nature become progressively transparent through the insights and actions of honest and consecrated men and women.[22] It is as people live in the light of the ideal here and now that

21   Stephen Lukes, 'Pathologies of Markets and States', *Miliband Lecture*, 16 March 2006, http://www.lse.ac.uk/collections/LSEPublicLecturesAndEvents/pdf/20060316-Lukes.pdf. Accessed 16 January 2007.
22   In this regard Oman comes close to the idea of praxis as it was developed by Marx and taken up by later thinkers.

they discover an 'intercourse with a greatness which admits of no finality, but requires absoluteness of loyalty both in seeking to know and to serve its ever expanding requirements'.[23]

It is, in particular, the commitment of people to act in terms of their insights into truth, goodness and beauty that, for Oman, brings about the transformation of the natural. There is a pattern here of change in response to new insights, which leads on in its turn to fresh insight and further change. Another way of seeing this is to say that there is a continual refreshing of the vision of what the divine requires of us. One possible example of what Oman is talking about here is the emancipation of slaves in the nineteenth century. The struggle for the emancipation of slaves was treated by many within the abolitionist movement as a 'high and sacred endeavour'.[24] It reflected an understanding of the sacred value of every human being. This understanding is now commonplace, though perhaps described in other terms; it is a 'secure achievement'. The attainment of this insight inspires Christians to fix the mark higher and wider out, such that, with this real insight into the sacred realm, there is a demand to go further in pursuing the 'infinite and eternal'.[25] A practical example of this might be the desire of some nineteenth-century radicals to link the abolition of slavery with the widening of the franchise. Another contemporary example might be the connections that some draw between the emancipation of slaves and just treatment for homosexuals. In this way, argues Oman, progress in the knowledge of the supernatural comes about through the attempt to transform that which is, the visible, in the light of the ideal, the supernatural. Religious knowledge is not gained through the acceptance or rejection of the natural, but by the natural becoming progressively diaphanous of the spiritual.[26]

Oman's idea of the 'natural' conveys the sense that creation is in a continual state of transition. Through human participation in God's

---

23   Oman, *The Natural and the Supernatural*, p.337.
24   See for instance Olaudad Equiano, *The Interesting Narrative and Other Writings* (Harmondsworth: Penguin, 2003). Equiano argues that the liberation of slaves is an aspect of their dignity as creatures made in the image of God.
25   Oman, *The Natural and the Supernatural*, p.338.
26   Ibid., p.338.

will, the world, rather than being ontologically static, is always in a process of 'becoming'. In principle, this transition includes a growth in knowledge, social evolution and physical change, and one can argue that this will include such changes as are offered by bio-scientific developments. Oman's framework provides, therefore, a context in which bioscience can be welcomed as one of the ways in which human beings are sharing with God in evolution. Evaluation of specific developments in bioscience will always be necessary, but a flexible and future-orientated view of nature prevents the theological panics associated with 'posthumanism': the perception that 'nature' is not fixed makes the notion that there are clear boundaries in the relationship between science and the human self/body problematic. Oman's work questions the distinction, crucial to a number of writers, between amelioration and transformation, which is, anyhow, rather arbitrary given the incremental nature of scientific progress.[27]

Sincerity

In his discussion of how it is that we, as individuals, can relate well to the supernatural, Oman stresses not only praxis, the practical out-working of one's insights, but also 'honesty' or 'sincerity'. In this regard Oman takes the poet as an exemplar of honesty. The poet, for Oman, is marked not only by a developed sensuousness, but also by 'aesthetic sincerity', where aesthetic refers to the 'response of feeling to all experience of environment'.[28] Aesthetic sincerity is exhibited through the poet's 'objective, unrestricted, unflinching facing of every kind of feeling, and all it revealed'.[29] In Oman's view the poet's sincerity involves putting whims and fancies to one side in order to focus on representing the world as it is experienced, without dis-

---

27   See for instance Brent Waters, *From Human to Posthuman: Christian Theology and Technology in a Postmodern World* (Aldershot: Ashgate, 2006).

28   Oman, *The Natural and the Supernatural*, p.126.

29   Ibid., p.127.

simulation or deception. Such an intention requires a great deal of courage involving, as it does, the eschewing of 'average opinions or conventionalities'.[30] The courage of the poet arises from a love of truth and is expressed in the desire to present human experience with all its stresses. Thus, for instance, the note of melancholy that is found in many of Shakespeare's works expresses his sense of the darker themes that colour the symphony of life.

One dimension of the sincerity that marks 'moral personality' is the recognition of the provisionality of all human knowledge. To live autonomously is to courageously recognise the uncertainty of one's grasp of the ideal, of truth, beauty and goodness. Contrawise, a typical form that insincerity takes is the pusillanimous search for finalities: fixed organisations, ethical schemes or theologies. The desire here is to avoid the insecurities of life; it is the search for security in an insecure world. In Oman's view, honesty forbids the postulation of finalities, but 'perhaps the sad story of man's whole history is that he would rather "have bondage with ease than strenuous liberty" and that this is just what life is appointed to disturb'.[31] To set up finalities is to attempt to avoid the difficult challenges posed by the human environment: 'to regard our opinions and practices as sacred is indeed the only quite impenetrable barricade against the assaults of chastening experience'.[32]

It is an interesting paradox that those who criticise bioscience as leading towards posthumanism and, in particular, the attempt to transcend human finitude, are also those who seem to claim some finality of insight into what it is to be human. One might have thought that an emphasis on human finitude would have coexisted with the recognition of epistemic limitation in the matter of ontology. It could be argued that it is an evolutionary perspective such as Oman's, which pays proper regard to the provisionality of human knowledge and the need to extend insight through careful attention to human experience, which, in point of fact, gives due weight to human finitude! The ways and will of God are discovered, for Oman, through careful attention to

30   Ibid., p.131.
31   John Oman, *Honest Religion* (Cambridge: CUP, 1941), p.40.
32   Oman, *The Natural and the Supernatural*, p.75.

experience rather than in a text or set practice. The texts and practices of the church are there to provide attitudinal orientation for the Christian, not a compendium of authoritative judgements.

Three implications for theological bioethics of Oman's experimental method may be mentioned. First, his emphasis on learning from experience means that ethics must be flexible and open to new insight. Second, it will be concerned to form judgements that arise from detailed scrutiny of scientific developments and the actual clinical use that these are put to. Third, theological ethics needs to work with an empirically realistic model of human experience, which moves beyond seeing human beings as analogous to a computational machine in which certain inputs draw forth necessary outcomes. Human existence, in actual fact, is typically marked by the holding together of apparently diverse and even contradictory emotions, desires, ends and values, and ethical judgements need to take this into account. For instance, it will not do to argue against PGD by claiming that 'selection' leads inevitably to a parent–child relationship characterised by instrumentality.

The benefits of forming ethical judgements on the basis of close scrutiny of scientific developments and actual clinical situations can be illustrated in relation to PGD. Jones outlines five possible uses of PGD: selection and implantation on the basis of viability; selection to exclude harmful genes, for instance, those responsible for cystic fibrosis; selection to exclude a gene likely to cause illness in later adult life; selection to determine sex; and selection to manipulate and design embryos so that they have certain desirable biological characteristics.[33] Consideration of these varied scenarios suggests that there are several issues pertinent to moral evaluation. One is the therapeutic value of the procedure in each case. Another is the question of whether there is coercion involved. A third is whether the scenarios are scientifically realistic. On this point, Jones argues that the last scenario lies in the realm of science fiction. Even if the technology were available to do the intricate gene therapy envisaged – which it will not be in the foreseeable future – the scenario takes no account of

33   Jones, 'Is PGD a Form of Eugenics?'

the complex interaction of the physical and the social in forming a person's intellectual and physical endowments.

Attention to actual developments and clinical practice suggest that there are no easy or unambiguous answers to ethical dilemmas, and this, I am arguing, is a view that is consistent with the adoption of an approach to bioethics such as that implied by Oman.

Conclusion

This chapter has explored Oman's work with a view to its relevance to bioethical discussions. An important aspect of Oman's theological anthropology is his emphasis on human autonomy as intrinsically worthwhile and extrinsically the means by which God's will for the world is revealed and actualised. Oman's work, it has been argued, highlights autonomy as an important theological value that Christians will wish to affirm in bioethical debates, though the ascription of dignity to the embryo suggests that autonomy cannot be an overriding ethical end.

Bioscientists may find theologians broadly encouraging or reactionary. A determinative issue will be the theological reading of 'nature'. Oman sees 'nature' as being a fluid, not a static, concept. It describes the current state of human knowledge and practice, but since recent experience has been of a cumulative growth in knowledge, moral and scientific, it follows that 'nature' is continually and rightly being revised. Moreover the revision of 'nature' is, for Oman, an expression of the will of God. This is a view that affirms technical and clinical progress, though not uncritically. It implies that God's will only emerges in the course of engaging closely and honestly with the bewildering mixture of theological ideas, legitimate ends, technical possibilities and actual clinical practice.

ANN MARIE MEALEY

The Bioethical Conscience

Introduction

When we hear expressions such as 'follow your heart', 'let conscience be your guide', or 'the truth lies within your heart', we are using the language of morality and of moral decision making. Although we may not be aware of the moral significance of such statements, we are aware that there is an element of moral decision making that lies within the heart of the individual and is shaped by their worldview and identity. This means that in the search for moral truth, we are not simply acting autonomously in any absolutist sense, or that our self-understanding and moral capabilities are derived *ex nihilo*; rather, we must acknowledge that our identity, self-understanding and moral worldview impinge on our moral choices. If, for instance, we view human life as sacred, created by God for God's purpose, this may shape the kind of arguments we might contribute to the contemporary debates concerning human genetics, stem cell research, eugenics, and the human genome project. If, on the other hand, we believe, for instance, that the human embryo is merely a cluster of cells with the potential for life and therefore not worthy of the status of a 'human person', then our stance on various biomedical issues may be quite different. We might conclude more easily that genetic manipulation of embryonic stem cells is not a violation of human dignity, and is therefore permissible in every instance.

This suggests that, although most of us would agree that having a moral conscience is important if we are to live a good life or to flourish as human beings, our conscience can lead us to different conceptions of the good, especially in new areas of ethical concern such as the human genome project or embryo experimentation. Tensions between religious believers' understanding of human life and that of secularists or humanists can lead to difficulties in discerning the truth about human genetics, enhancement, embryonic stem cells, the status of the dead human body, or eugenic interventions of any kind. Indeed, claims made by a magisterial teaching authority may further exacerbate tensions in these arenas, by demanding conformity to its guidelines, without ensuring that members of the faithful are fully informed about the complexities of assessing bioethical matters. Policy makers can also confuse things by making decisions that do not consider minority or religious views.

Further problems which need to be considered when discussing the role of what I am going to call the 'bioethical conscience' pertain to the lack of transparency in some areas of bioethics, which leads to suspicion about the kinds of experimentations and practices that scientists are promoting in the so-called attempt to enhance human life and cure disease. This often leads to a breakdown in dialogue between people, and makes the possibility of having an 'informed conscience' seem unrealistic, or, worse, marginalises those who do not conform to the predominant consensus. That there is a need to reflect more closely on the nature and role of our moral conscience in bioethical matters is clear. In order to do this, however, we need first to be clear about what we mean by the term 'moral conscience', and then distinguish the adult or informed conscience from the infantile one.

What is Conscience?

Although its definition is often vague, when we speak about moral conscience there is an acknowledgement that it relates in some way to deeply held moral convictions.[1] It is considered as the means through which human persons discern good from evil and choose actions that express their inner convictions. In this sense, it involves a certain degree of self-awareness and self-education. Obeying one's conscience

---

1   Linda Hogan, *Confronting the Truth: Conscience and the Catholic Tradition* (London: Darton, Longman & Todd, 2000), p.9.

is not simply a matter of following feelings or desires for reasons of self-interest or fear; rather, having a mature moral conscience carries with it the burden of seeking the truth in a way that does not reduce moral actions to mere conformity, obedience to authority for its own sake, or for social or religious convention. Moral agents have a responsibility to acquire and to understand relevant moral principles, and then to know how these are to be applied in the light of their internal convictions.[2]

The notion of conscience carries with it the understanding that all human persons have the *capacity* (even if they choose not to use it, or cannot use it because of fear, ignorance, or some psychological reason) to determine their own lives in freedom. This belief is not simply a secular one. *The Catechism of the Catholic Church*, for example, states that, as we are human beings created in the image and likeness of God, we are capable of directing ourselves towards genuine goodness. (n.1704ff.) The Catholic theologian William May explains that:

> Human persons, created in the image and likeness of God, have the power of free choice. In order to create a being to whom he could give his own life, God created persons (angelic and human) who have the power to make or break their own lives by their own free choices.[3]

Gaudium et Spes, one of the documents of Vatican II, states that:

> Deep within their conscience men and women discover a law which they have not laid upon themselves and which they must obey. Its voice, ever calling them to love and to do what is good and to avoid evil, tells them inwardly at the right moment: do this, shun that. For they have in their hearts a law inscribed by God. (*GS* 16)

More recently, the inviolability of conscience has been emphasised in the Papal Encyclical, *Veritatis Splendor*, where John Paul II affirms

---

2   Patrick Hannon, *Knowing Right from Wrong: Thoughts from the Catechism of the Catholic Church* (Dublin: Veritas, 1995), p.23.
3   William E. May, *An Introduction to Moral Theology* (Indiana: Sunday Publishing Division, 1994), p.26.

that conscience is the link between human freedom and moral truth. The relationship between freedom and God's law, he explains, is 'most deeply lived out in the "heart" of the person, in his moral conscience'. (*VS* 54)

It is clear that conscience has a special place in the hearts and minds of religious believers as well as humanists. Insofar as it refers to our capacity to choose good over evil and live a good life in freedom, it is a human phenomenon, not merely a religious one. None the less, the concept of conscience is not without its difficulties, one of which involves differentiating between the mature conscience and the infantile one. As human beings, we are vulnerable; and sometimes our vulnerability makes us fearful that unless we conform to the expectations and guidelines of an authority figure, we shall lose something, perhaps approval or praise. On other occasions we conform because we just do not possess the necessary information to make an informed judgement. We rely on the opinion or counsel of an authority or a significant other to make the decision for us. Indeed, we may even be fearful that if we follow our moral conscience, we will be marginalised from our churches or communities because we do not share the predominant consensus. As Richard Gula puts it, 'we regulate our behaviour so as not to lose love and approval. As a matter of self-protection, we absorb the standards and regulations of our parents, or anyone who has authority over us.'[4] In other words, our conscience is often reduced to the infantile conscience, conforming out of a fear of loss of love from an institution, community, or authority figure.

When this happens, it is often difficult to see how one could begin to conceive of individuals being able to assess independently the ethical issues presented to us by the field of genetics. How do we know that we are really following our conscience if we do not know the full facts about the issues? Who should tell us? When we make judgements about eugenics, are we really acting in freedom when we are scarcely able to comprehend the scientific data? Should we follow our tradition if all else fails? Where should we obtain the necessary information for us to make sound moral judgements, and to ensure

4   Richard Gula, 'Conscience', in *Christian Ethics: An Introduction*, ed. Bernard Hoose (London: Cassell, 1988), p.111.

that we are really acting in freedom and not out of fear or ignorance? Can we dissent from the dominant consensus point of view? Is the religious perspective an acceptable one? Are Christians vulnerable in the face of a scientific worldview?

The Informed Conscience and Bioethics

In order to attempt to answer some of these questions, we must first be clear about what we mean by the term 'informed conscience'. This will help us to understand more clearly how and in what way our conscience is educated and how it needs intellectual (scientific) elements as well as affective ones.

Although conscience is generally spoken of as the expression of a person's identity and/or perspective, it is important to break it down into conceptual categories so that we can see more clearly what constitutes this identity. Since conscience involves the individual coming to a decision on a particular issue, it includes not only the individual's story, background, experiences, environment and feelings, but also their attitudinal, intellectual and somatic aspects as well. To use Richard Gula's turn of phrase, conscience is 'me coming to a decision'.[5] In this respect, conscience involves a person at their deepest level, and its expression often gives us a glimpse of the character of a person, or of the kind of values, or commitment to values, that they possess.

For Timothy O'Connell, there are three categories of conscience, known respectively as conscience 1, conscience 2 and conscience 3.[6] Although distinct, these senses or dimensions of conscience interact at various stages in our moral development and impact on our moral behaviour. Conscience 1 (also known as *synderesis*) is perhaps the

5   Richard Gula, *Reason Informed by Faith: Foundations of Catholic Morality* (New York: Paulist Press, 1989), p.131.
6   Timothy O'Connell, *Principles for A Catholic Morality* (New York: Seabury Press, 1978), pp.52–53.

easiest to describe, as it refers to our capacity to know the good. This is an orientation which all human beings are believed to possess and which gives us our fundamental, and frequently unique, stance towards the world, good and evil, right and wrong. However, having a 'sense' of what is right is not sufficient; conscience 1 needs to be educated and developed so that our moral responses are not the result of mere speculation, subjective preference, selfishness or the desire for power.

The shortcomings of conscience 1 show that we need to have a more scientific and objective element to our moral reasoning. It is not enough simply to follow our sense of the good; we need to educate our conscience in the art of right reasoning, balanced decision making, and sound judgement. We need to examine the nature of moral principles, the values that our tradition proposes to us, the guidance of our parents, relevant scientific data, as well as the moral guidelines proposed to us by figures of authority. It is not simply the case that we should follow these rules or moral proposals blindly; conscience 2 expects us to know *why* we are choosing a particular course of action over another. It demands of us that we understand the moral significance of our actions. This is what is often referred to as 'moral science', because it is defined as the 'the process of discovering the particular good which ought to be done or the evil to be avoided'.[7]

It is in this category that we would place any religious values or the sources of moral wisdom of a particular religious tradition or magisterium. The texts and stories of one's tradition can also be considered to be a source of moral wisdom in the sense that, as Paul Ricoeur explains, they allow us to 'relate goodness with happiness and evil with unhappiness'.[8] Very often, the foundational stories of good and evil of our communities are the means through which we gain a heightened sense of what the good life entails. The significance of these stories lies in their ability to give us a sense of belonging as we search for truth, as well as providing us with an imaginative space in

7   Gula, *Reason Informed by Faith*, p.131.
8   Paul Ricoeur, *Time and Narrative I*, trans. Kathleen Blamey, Kathleen McLoughlin and David Pellauer (Chicago and London: University of Chicago Press, 1984), p.40.

which we can try out various proposals for living. By following the development of characters in stories, we come to know the kinds of character traits necessary for moral growth, virtue and maturity.

More importantly, perhaps, the narratives of one's community allow the moral agent to recognise and describe the virtues in a symbolic, rather than an abstract, way. Narrative fleshes out the contours of the virtues which would be all but incomprehensible without stories to explain their meaning. 'To understand what courage means, we tell the story of Achilles; to understand what wisdom means, we tell the story of St Francis of Assisi.'[9] This is important for the development of moral conscience because it makes us aware that truth is not derived *ex nihilo* and that our tradition can help to sustain us as we search for truth. Following one's conscience is not simply a matter of ignoring tradition or the received wisdom of one's community; rather, it involves reflecting on these in a deep and meaningful way in order to find the path of righteousness.

This clearly shows that conscience 2 (moral science) is a complex category of conscience that draws upon many sources of moral wisdom for its development. Depending on the ways in which individuals combine the various strands of their lives together in some cohesive form, the decisions a person will take might vary considerably. This is the case because it is at this stage (conscience 2) that our perceptions of the good are formed and interact with the environment in which we find ourselves. So, for example, religious believers may find themselves grappling not only with what the scientific field has to say about human life, but also with what the magisterial teaching authority and the Bible have to say about human life, healing, suffering, disease, IVF, eugenics, or bioethics. The sources of moral wisdom may often conflict, and there may be lively disagreement about what is right and what is wrong, but it is important to note that when an individual acts, it is an expression of all the various strands of their life coming together. This shows that the self should be understood in a hermeneutical way (that is, in a way that acknowledges that

9   Richard Kearney, *On Paul Ricoeur: The Owl of Minerva*, Transcending the Boundaries in Philosophy and Theology Series (Aldershot: Ashgate, 2004), p.114.

our lives are a complex web of stories, experiences, and identities) as well as paying due regard to the fact that the self and meaning in any sense is a *project* – a desire to be, a process of interpretation that can never be completed in any total sense.[10]

This recognition of the need to understand the self as a process is central to understanding the relationship of Christian ethics to bio-ethical debate. It facilitates a receptive openness towards the complex phenomena which bear on moral decision making: the biblical story, moral experience, culture, magisterium, and community. Acknowledgement of the dialectic character of moral decision making from both a religious and a secular stance means that we do not presume to have all the answers in advance of the process of interpretation of, and reflection upon, the sources of moral wisdom that we draw upon for help and guidance. Of course, not having all the answers makes the process of discernment all the more complex and tedious but, when individuals search for truth in this way, they are more likely to notice when their moral decision making is being manipulated by others for whatever reason.

Despite the complexities involved in the education of our moral conscience, most of us do move from perception to action. The interaction of conscience 1 with conscience 2 is a complex process, the results of which depend on the interplay of a range of factors which the individual must assess, but it does lead to a judgement – a judgement of what must be done now and a commitment to seeing it through. What is significant here is that no one can make this judgement for the individual; it is something we must choose for ourselves, in the hope that our conscience will lead us to what is true and just. Each judgement of conscience, therefore, comprises 'the person's best

---

10   This idea is derived from Paul Ricoeur's interpretation of tradition as being both closed to preserve the wisdom of the past and open to ensure that new perspectives and interpretations of tradition are possible. For a detailed account of Ricoeur's position, see Paul Ricoeur, *Time and Narrative III*, pp.220–27. For a simple and clear statement of Ricoeur's position on tradition and history see Christian Delacroix, 'De quelques usages historiens de P. Ricoeur', in Bertrand Müller, *L'Histoire entre mémoire et épistemologie: Autour de Paul Ricoeur* (Lausanne: Éditions Payot, 2005), pp.99–123.

and truthful estimation of goodness in a given situation. They are held with integrity and involve an obligation to carry them through.'[11]

The Bioethical Conscience

While there is undoubtedly an element of self-determination involved in 'following one's conscience', it is important to stress that this self-determination (conscience 3) is subject to, and dependent upon, conscience 2. This means that, in order to make a truthful decision about, say, IVF, experimentation on embryos, or stem cell research, the individual is required to possess and to assess relevant data, including that of a scientific nature, before making a decision. Conscience 2 requires an ability to justify our moral positions rationally, and to make decisions that arise from a genuine and sincere attempt to engage not only with one's worldview or tradition, but also with any new data that might be of relevance to our ethical assessment of, for example, procuring embryonic stem cells in order to cure disease.

This can be difficult for the non-scientific, non-academic individual. It seems to me that many of the debates in the field of bioethics require such a high level of expertise that the ordinary person who wishes to seek the truth may find it difficult to claim with any great certainty that they are informed about bioethical issues. For instance, the distinction that Gareth Jones makes in this volume between therapeutic and enhancement procedures is significant for Christians believers who feel that, owing to the fact that it goes beyond what is necessary to sustain or restore good health, any form of enhancement is morally wrong. Jones argues that there are categories of enhancement that ought to be acceptable to Christian believers by virtue of the fact that they are 'variations of therapy, even though ... by current standards highly technological variants'.[12] These latter refer to cases

11   Hogan, *Confronting the Truth*, p.12.
12   D. Gareth Jones, 'Enhancement: Is Baseless Speculation Misleading Theologians and Bioethicists?', this volume, p.130.

where, through the genetic manipulation of embryos, Alzheimer's or coronary disease could be treated. This would not make the individual person superhuman, nor interfere with any of their capabilities; rather, it would perform a more therapeutic function and improve the life expectancy and quality of life of that individual.

Of course, one could ask whether tolerance and/or acceptance of such a limited use of embryos might provide a gateway for other more unacceptable or abusive applications, but it is also important to stress that, in order to assess the ethical significance of this type of enhancement, individuals need to be fully informed. Without an adequate grasp of the procedures involved in bioethical issues, how can any individual claim to know the truth, or defend a particular point of view? And given that we are all called to be moral by virtue of being human, is it not, therefore, imperative that the bioethical debates are not confined to the academic and scientific arena, and that the language of bioethics is made accessible to the non-specialist?

The risk of being 'kept in the dark' about bioethical matters is that individuals will be unable to claim that they are following their conscience in any real way. They will just follow a rule or principle, analogous to the way in which one would follow the law, out of fear of disapproval from an authority, simply because they did not know what else to do. While this could help policy makers and church leaders to defend a particular point of view more forcefully, by claiming that most members of society accept it without question, it could also increase the chances of individuals being coerced rather than informed about the various issues involved in the field of bioethics.

Genuine moral living comes not from blind obedience but from a sincere engagement with the varied facets of human existence. It may be the case that an individual's conscience will coincide with the authority in question, or with the law, but what is important is that the decision is the result of the individual's commitment to doing and finding the truth, not from a fear of retribution, exclusion from a community, or disapproval of some sort. One possible way to ensure that individuals are informed is, perhaps, to set up local information services or parish support groups that could advise and educate their members about the facts, using non-specialist language, and hence enourage a contrite engagement with the issues and a commitment to seeking the truth, rather than merely speculating about it.

Whose Bioethics?

The success or failure of such attempts will undoubtedly depend upon the willingness of practitioners and those in positions of power to provide honest and transparent accounts of bioethical procedures and practices and to listen to alternative, including minority, points of view. Frequently, individuals feel marginalised when 'one version of bioethics becomes predominant, and its practitioners attain positions of influence and power in government, academic and professional circles'.[13] This makes following a different path – in conscience – quite difficult, especially when those in power seek to work with and converse with only those individuals who will help them to promote the dominant agenda. This is known as 'consensus building'. When this happens, the resulting 'consensus' or opinion is not one that has been reached in genuine conscience but one that has been adopted by like-minded people.[14] There is then little room for minority views or genuine debate and exchanges of opinions between individuals and communities, religious or otherwise.

If after attempting to engage with the relevant facts of a bio-ethical procedure, an individual, perhaps for religious reasons, decides not to conform to the dominant consensus, they should not be dismissed as being irrational or insignificant. Questioning the dominant consensus can often lead our conscience more deeply towards the truth, because we are not simply seeking to promote one particular agenda, political or otherwise, or to conform to societal pressure. Rather, we are offering an honest and sincere account of the good as we perceive it. This kind of questioning can lead to a process of

13   Sean Murphy, 'Establishment Bioethics', http://www.consciencelaws.org/ Examining-Conscience-Ethical/Ethical 16.html, p.2. Accessed 9 October 2006.
14   Ibid.

'unmasking', or to a hermeneutics of suspicion, which might prevent us from merely accepting a consensus out of fear or because we believe that an alternative position will not be tolerated or will be deemed unorthodox. As Paul Ricoeur asserts, far from undermining orthodoxy, questioning received wisdom or 'presumed truth' gives rise to and facilitates a more orthodox version of truth.[15]

This is the case because, when we question received wisdom in the light of new phenomena or new information, it ensures that this wisdom continues to inform our ethical judgements and that our traditions are truly living and representative of how we should live and act today. Indeed, influenced by the work of Jürgen Habermas, Ricoeur argues further that the truths of tradition *must* be summoned to the tribunal of critique and suspicion in order to be evaluated for its authenticity. Tradition and our notion of received wisdom need to be unmasked and scrutinised so that our notion of truth and/or tradition does not consist in accepting the ideologies of interest groups who are in power. This type of healthy questioning is necessary because authorities may well distort our vision of ourselves, or of the good, for their own political or ideological gain.[16]

It is equally important to note here, however, that without some guidance from a magisterium or recognised authority, we are more at risk of following cultural trends, fashions or subcultures. Although conscience cannot be formed by an external authority, equally it cannot proceed to make sound ethical judgements without the help of an authority of some sort. This indicates that the process of following one's conscience, in genetics and in all other areas of human life, will always exist in the tension between what is proposed by tradition and

15   Paul Ricoeur, *Time and Narrative III*, trans. Kathleen Blamey, Kathleen McLoughlin and David Pellauer (Chicago and London: University of Chicago Press, 1988), p.222. Here Ricoeur explains that distancing ourselves from the dominant consensus or from tradition allows us to 'sift through the dead traditions in which we no longer recognise ourselves'.

16   Paul Ricoeur, *From Text to Action*: *Essays in Hermeneutics II*, trans. Kathleen Blamey and John B. Thompson (Evanston, Illinois: Northwestern University Press, 1991), pp.284ff. See also Graeme Nicholson, 'Answers to Critical Theory', in *Gadamer and Hermeneutics*, Continental Philosophy IV, edited and with an introduction by Hugh J. Silverman (London: Routledge, 1991), p.158.

what our conscience tends to lead us towards. At times, both of these will guide us towards the same ethical stance, but they will also lead to debate and to dialogue, which may require revision of opinion and further reflection. This dialogue need not be interpreted in a negative light, for it is only in the creative tension between self, society, tradition, science, faith and reason that we can be assured that our moral responses are the result of a genuine engagement with who we think we are and what we think is representative of truth. No one should feel vulnerable in the search for meaning and understanding, as we are all called, whether religious or otherwise, to seek the truth about genetics and to ask about the value of human life in our contemporary age.

Nevertheless, this dialogue can only take place if we are adequately informed about the issues that are facing us in this age of genetics and if we can be assured that the institutions in which we trust for guidance and support, both religious and secular, provide us with truthful information and facilitate genuine dialogue and debate (rather than demanding conformity) so that our consciences will lead us to the truth in love. As St Paul tells us: 'when we sin against the members of [our human] family, and wound their conscience when it is weak, [we] sin against Christ.' (1 Corinthians 8:10)

Part Two: Moral Boundaries

D. GARETH JONES AND MAJA I. WHITAKER

Scientific Fraud: The Demise of Idealistic Science

Introduction

From a vantage point in the 1950s one would have found it difficult to believe that fifty years hence scientific endeavour would have become embroiled in fraud. In the 1950s and 1960s the scientific community was still reeling from the Piltdown fraud, which stood out as a cause celebre. Whilst this might not have been a unique event, its effect reverberated down through the years, and scientific careers (even posthumously) were still being besmirched decades later. This was because science was viewed as the epitome of honesty and integrity. It was indeed the means of uncovering what some regarded as objective truth. This objectivity stemmed from its apparent lack of interpretive biases, undergirded by the honesty of its practitioners. This set science apart from other approaches to reality, and placed it in the upper echelons of worldview hierarchies. Theology, in particular, was seen as contributing little, if anything, to what one could reliably know about the world; it was regarded as lacking in objectivity and possibly even honesty. Science could be relied upon; little else could.

Perhaps life was never this simple, and yet many of the advocates of scientific rationalism, the high priests one might say of scientific religiosity, saw scientific investigation as superior to all other forms of human endeavour. This is why scientific fraud was unimaginable, being little less than heresy and a relinquishing of science's moral authority.

Such descriptions must seem strange and idyllic to those brought up in a scientific environment characterised by high financial stakes, close associations with industry, research assessment exercises, alignment with the national good and economic imperatives. Science has indeed lost its innocence, and with this has come a change in its moral underpinnings. While fraud in science is, of course, frowned upon, its endemic presence within most scientific disciplines has revealed a disturbing moral flabbiness to the underbelly of the scientific establishment.

But where does this leave science? And how should Christians respond to science, especially in areas where it appears to be treading on theological and moral toes? Does the presence of fraud lead to the conclusion that science has lost any moral imperative and so is to be distrusted and opposed?

But why such widespread fraud? Is it due solely to the overweening ambition of frail scientists, or does the responsibility lie, at least in part, with the excessive demands placed upon science by society? Groups within our communities are desperate for scientific breakthroughs to remedy their personal tragedies, and this adds to the pressure on scientists to take short-cuts and even invent the data they would like to obtain.

Case Study: Stem Cell Research

The system within which scientists conduct research is a demanding one. It expects progress, rewarding scientists who demonstrate it and ignoring or censuring those who do not. The quantity and prestige of researchers' publications are used to evaluate their careers and often determine their professional advancement, creating a pressure to publish. Even small differences in publication output rates between scientists can translate into greatly differing rewards and recognition: 'those who publish more, earn more.'[1] Scientists often find themselves in a race for results as they compete with other researchers to publish first on a 'hot' topic. The fast pace at which biomedical science is progressing and the rapidity with which results are published online add to the rush.

1   R. Freeman, E. Weinstein, E. Marincola, J. Rosenbaum and F. Solomon, 'Competition and Careers in Biosciences', *Science* 294, 2001, pp.2293–94.

When the expected progress is not actually being made, the temptation is to manipulate appearances to make it seem as if it is, even if only to a small degree. Many researchers cut corners on their experiments, prioritising speed over quality.[2] Accusations have even been made that major journals themselves cut corners to publish the most prestigious papers.[3] Many researchers have admitted to their involvement in a range of mundane questionable behaviours that do not fit the definition of fabrication, falsification or plagiarism, but still threaten the integrity of scientific research.[4] When this behaviour is taken to the extreme, some researchers are found to have committed outright fraud. The case of Hwang Woo-Suk in South Korea provides an all-too-pertinent example.

The name of Hwang Woo-Suk has hit the headlines repeatedly over the last few years. In 2004 he became the first scientist to clone human embryos and extract stem cells from them, with a landmark paper in the very prestigious journal, *Science*.[5] As if that was not enough, in May 2005 his team announced (again in *Science*) the creation of the world's first embryonic stem cells using genetic material from patients,[6] and therefore matched to these individual

2   H. Pearson, 'It's a scoop!', *Nature* 426, 2003, pp.222−23.
3   D. Adam and H. Knight, 'Publish, and be damned ...', *Nature* 419, 2002, pp.772−76.
4   B. C. Martinson, M. S. Anderson and R. de Vries, 'Scientists behaving badly', *Nature* 435, 2005, pp.737−38.
5   W. S. Hwang, Y. J. Ryu, J. H. Park, E. S. Park, E. G. Lee, J. M. Koo, H. Y. Jeon, B. C. Lee, S. K. Kang, S. J. Kim, C. Ahn, J. H. Hwang, K. Y. Park, J. B. Cibelli and S. Y. Moon, 'Evidence of a pluripotent human embryonic stem cell line derived from a cloned blastocyst', *Science* 303, 2004, pp.1669−74.
6   W. S. Hwang, S. I. Roh, B. C. Lee, S. K. Kang, D. K. Kwon, S. Kim, S. J. Kim, S. W. Park, H. S. Kwon, C. K. Lee, J. B. Lee, J. M. Kim, C. Ahn, S. H. Paek, S. S. Chang, J. J. Koo, H. S. Yoon, J. H. Hwang, Y. Y. Hwang, Y. S. Park, S. K. Oh, H. S. Kim, J. H. Park, S. Y. Moon and G. Schatten, 'Patient-specific embryonic stem cells derived from human SCNT blastocysts', *Science* 308, 2005, pp.1777−83.

patients. He even went further with the birth of Snuppy, the world's first cloned dog, in August 2005.[7]

Taken together, the two landmark papers seemed to represent a scientific milestone. Therapeutic cloning, with its potential to produce replacement cells and tissues, had become a reality; cloning actually worked in humans. A whole new area of research had been shown to be feasible.

In the wake of all these exciting developments, a not-for-profit worldwide network for human embryo cloning was established (the World Stem Cell Hub), with the cloning work to be carried out in Korea and the resulting cell lines shipped around the world. The future for human embryonic stem cell research looked very rosy and enticing.

The plaudits came thick and fast – from across the world's scientific community, but mainly from South Korea. Hwang became a national hero, perhaps embarrassingly so. For instance, he was hailed as the 'supreme scientist' and, as is fitting for such a person, a postage stamp was dedicated to him. South Korea became the centre of human embryonic stem cell research, much to the chagrin of the United States as well as some other countries.

And then everything began to unravel. Ethical issues began to surface, since it appeared that two junior female members of Hwang's research group had donated their own eggs for use in the programme. Then there were suggestions that they may have been coerced into doing so. Had they provided truly informed consent? Hwang initially denied these allegations. But things were to get worse. At the end of 2005, an investigation into one of Hwang's collaborators revealed that up to 20 egg donors had been paid for providing their eggs (a painful procedure that can have serious side-effects). These revelations led to Hwang resigning as head of the World Stem Cell Hub.

Questions began to be asked. If a scientist is unethical in these ways, could he also have been unethical in the scientific work itself –

---

7   B. C. Lee, M. K. Kim, G. Jang, H. J. Oh, F. Yuda, H. J. Kim, M. H. Shamim, J. J. Kim, S. K. Kang, G. Schatten and W. S. Hwang, 'Dogs cloned from adult somatic cells', *Nature* 436, 2005, p.641.

in the ways in which the experiments had been conducted? Lack of integrity undermines the essence of science.

Unfortunately, the situation was in fact far worse than anyone could have imagined. Hwang had indeed fabricated just about everything (although Snuppy still remains a true clone). One ethicist has referred to this as a 'moral tsunami in the world of stem cell research', characterised by 'a very malodorous bag of smoke, lies and obfuscation'.[8] Hwang resigned from his post at Seoul National University. The scientific community and the general public have had to concede that they were duped for a while. Hwang was later dismissed.

Patriotism in science is always dangerous. Science is an international activity paying little regard to national or cultural boundaries. Scientific reputations are usually earned slowly and painstakingly, on the basis of sustained performance open to the scrutiny and probing analysis of one's peers. Hwang rapidly became little less than a 'rock star' of science, in a country eager to bestow such an accolade on one of its own. South Korea envisioned itself as an international leader in biotechnology – an ambitious plan for which Hwang was the poster boy. Whenever this is the case, enormous care has to be exercised, because science by its very nature challenges big names and big ideas. Science is more comfortable with critical analysis and the overthrowing of dogma than it is with instant fame.

Why did Hwang act as he did? Obviously we do not have an answer. But we can speculate that he may have surmised that someone else would come along quite soon and clone human embryos. In doing this, they would have thereby corroborated his (fraudulent, although quite reasonable) claims, and Hwang would have gained the credit by publishing first. The trouble is that he may have made the cloning of human embryos appear too easy. The reality appears to be that it is very difficult. A small number of groups in the United States, China[9]

---

8   A. Caplan, 'The end of stem cell research? Hardly', MSNBC, 3 January 2006. See http://www.msnbc.msn.com/id/10683107/. Accessed 27 March 2006.

9   Y. Chen, Z. X. He, A. Liu, K. Wang, W. W. Mao, J. X. Chu, Y. Lu, Z. F. Fang, Y. T. Shi, Q. Z. Yang, da Y. Chen, M. K. Wang, J. S. Li, S. L. Huang, X. Y. Kong, Y. Z. Shi, Z. Q. Wang, J. H. Xia, Z. G. Long, Z. G. Xue, W. X. Ding and H. Z. Sheng, 'Embryonic stem cells generated by nuclear transfer of human somatic nuclei into rabbit oocytes', *Cell Research* 13, 2003, pp.251–63.

and the United Kingdom[10] have produced human clones (blastocysts), although the clones have only survived for a few days, and stem cells have not, to date, been extracted from them. Whenever someone gives the impression that something like this is easy, they are probably wrong. It should also be borne in mind that the first claim that a human had been cloned (an actual breathing living individual) was made in 1978. On that occasion it was a journalistic hoax.[11,12,13] Cloning appears to lend itself to such claims, such is the glamour (and sometimes notoriety) attaching to it.

An editorial in the newspaper *Chosun Ilbo* has given five reasons why the fraudulent Hwang episode went undetected for such a long time. The first was the rigid hierarchical structure in Hwang's research team, by which Hwang controlled the careers of his colleagues. They followed orders, even deception and fraud. Second, the institutional ethics committee acted as little more than a rubber stamp. Thirdly, Hwang's papers had as many as 25 co-authors, who appeared to want to bask in the glory of their hero. Fourth, the government was more interested in providing Hwang with bodyguards, to protect its huge financial stake in the research, than with assuring the authenticity of the results. Fifthly, the media failed to act as a watchdog, instead promoting scientific commercialism and joining in with the excessive enthusiasm of everyone else.[14]

Scientific fraud is always tragic and self-defeating. It misleads other scientists, sending them down useless paths, thereby wasting money, time and energy. In leading research down blind alleys, it can

10   M. Stojkovic, P. Stojkovic, C. Leary, V. J. Hall, L. Armstrong, M. Herbert, M. Nesbitt, M. Lako and A. Murdoch, 'Derivation of a human blastocyst after heterologous nuclear transfer to donated oocytes', *Reproductive Biomedicine Online* 11, 2005, pp.226–31.
11   D. M. Rorvik, *In His Image* (Melbourne: Nelson, 1978).
12   B. J. Culliton, 'Scientists dispute book's claim that human clone has been born', *Science* 199, 1978, pp.1314–16.
13   W. J. Broad, 'Court affirms: boy clone saga is a hoax', *Science* 213, 1981, pp.118–19.
14   Editorial, 'Woo-Suk Hwang: Case Closed', *Chosun Ilbo*, 12 May 2006. See http://english.chosun.com/w21data/html/news/200605/200605120035.html. Accessed 9 June 2006.

close off potentially fruitful areas of research. It ruins careers: in this case, it was not just Hwang's, but many of those in his team and even in other teams pursuing similar goals. It creates expectations on the part of patients who hope to benefit from the fruits of research, because it suggests that we have abilities we do not possess. It is said that 14,000 people had registered with the World Stem Cell Hub, hoping for cures for spinal cord and other injuries. This is nothing less than appalling deception. In the eyes of some, it even undermines the integrity of the whole of the scientific endeavour. But, in the end, those who are fraudulent nearly always get found out. Even the most acclaimed results require independent validation before they are truly accepted.

We should not expect science to move too rapidly. That has been a major problem in the whole area of therapeutic (research) cloning. Scientists closely involved in mammalian cloning, let alone human cloning, know the pitfalls. It is very slow and very difficult. The trouble with Hwang is that he probably got caught up in the excessive hype and expectations, leading him to cut corners and then deliberately fabricate results. His results were all too quickly accepted by a world eager for progress. It has been explained that: 'As the demand for results far outstripped the ability of researchers to supply them, a seller's market emerged in which goods were overvalued and even low-quality merchandise was snatched up by eager buyers.'[15] What needs to be learnt from this is that science does not advance in predictable ways. Neither does it advance according to the time schedules of the media or politicians. Impatient scientists may attempt to put the research machine into overdrive, but the inevitable complexity of the task causes some to push the moral rather than the scientific boundaries to produce the expected results.

15   D. A. Shaywitz, 'Stem Cell Hype and Hope', *Washington Post*, 12 January 2006, A21.

Why should we take Fraud seriously?

Fraud overturns the truthfulness of science

Truth and honesty are the essence of science; the scientific endeavour itself comprises a search for truth, even if it is truth within a very restricted framework. This search must be conducted with a spirit of honesty and openness, without which the endeavour is self-defeating. In this spirit, scientists are generally motivated by a drive for precision and objectivity, a drive that is essential for the elaboration of new scientific concepts. Truth and honesty go hand in hand, and without them science loses both its authority and its power.

In overturning the truthfulness of science, fraud undermines its very essence. There is no such thing as deceptive science; if it is deceptive it is not science. Research that produces poor, unrepeatable results, or that proposes hypotheses incapable of being tested, is the antithesis of science and is valueless. Though such sloppy science may not be fraudulent, it can have similar consequences. Science that does not lead to reliable data is robbed of practical power. This is amply demonstrated in the biomedical sciences, where inflated hopes are cynically betrayed and expectations of cures vanish into the gloom of deceit.

Hwang's fraudulent results and grand promises served to raise the hopes of thousands of desperately ill patients. All over the world, patients watched with great anticipation as he trumpeted his success in the media and established the World Stem Cell Hub. But with the deception exposed, these hopes have been dashed, or at the least diminished to more realistic proportions.[16] In other words, when scientists cut corners, or deliberately fabricate results, the repercussions extend far beyond scientific advancement or their own reputations.

The truth and honesty lying at the heart of genuine scientific investigations point to the Christian declaration that these values are

16   B. Demick, 'Faith in "Miracle Cures" is Fading in South Korea', *Los Angeles Times*, 5 March 2006. Available at: http://www.latimes.com/news/nationworld/world/la-fg-stemcell5mar05,1,5197240.story. Accessed 27 March 2006.

integral to the basic structure of God's world. This is why Christian and scientific aspirations have so much in common, since both reflect different facets of the same truth. Fraud and deception are foreign to both, and undermine both.

Christians, therefore, should be the first to defend the significance of these values in science, and to abhor pressures that militate against them. It is not my intention to probe these pressures, except to say that they stem from the increasingly close association between governments and commercial interests in university research.

Fraud is the antithesis of servanthood

Fraud has its basis in the desire to be first; to be pre-eminent; to be number one. However, in order to attain this status, people are prepared to dominate others, and to trick them. It is lying and falsehood. Much about the drive to acquire prestige is not confined to science; it is something we encounter in every area of life. And yet in a way it is endemic to the scientific endeavour, since science in its modern guise is highly competitive and status driven.

This is readily demonstrated when we think of the names of scientists that live on from one year to the next, or even one generation to the next. Most people have little difficulty in remembering the name of the first surgeon to carry out a heart transplant, Christiaan Barnard, but no recollection of the second person, Norman Shumway. The reality, however, is that some of these 'also rans' did far more ground-breaking work and careful studies on heart transplantation. It was this work which set the scene for the ultimate long-term success of this procedure, even though most of the work was conducted far away from the media spotlight. The Christian aphorism that comes most readily to mind is that 'the first shall be last, and the last shall be first'. (Matthew 20:16)

The drive to be first must be curbed if we are to live with the Christian priorities of humility and servanthood. We are called to serve others, to work for their good, putting our energy and skills towards their interests rather than our own. (Philippians 2:3–4) The temptation to seek the limelight or to be honoured as the first or best must be withstood. Instead, we should ask what will serve others and advance their interests. This frequently requires us to put aside personal prestige and to collaborate with others, working together for the common good.

This provides the most congenial environment for scientific activity, although it is all too readily undermined. Collaboration and learning from others, accepting the contribution of those with complementary techniques and ideas at their disposal; all this is inherent within much successful science. This is the positive face of the large research groups that spearhead so much of today's ground-breaking science. While most of those involved in these groups would not think of them in terms of servanthood, they certainly reflect the importance of community effort.

However, such groups can be poisoned by the fraud of just one member. The whole edifice comes tumbling down, and the group effort is irremediably destroyed by the deception of one person. The tragedy is easy to see, and reminds us of the need for openness, integrity and honesty on the part of all. Hwang's fraud brought one career after another to an end, as the members of his team have suffered irreparable harm.

Fraud leads to poor stewardship

At a practical level, fraud leads to poor stewardship; it is simply wasteful. Hwang appears to have wasted money and resources. He had received multi-million dollar funding from the South Korean government and private donors for his cloning work, some of which he has been charged with embezzling.[17] It has also been revealed that Hwang had received more than 2000 donated eggs, approximately five times the figure that had been acknowledged in his published

17   C. Sang-Hun, 'South Korean scientist indicted in cloning scandal', *International Herald Tribune*, 12 May 2006. See http://www.iht.com/articles/2006/05/12/news/korea.php. Accessed 25 May 2006.

papers.[18] The use of these eggs for ultimately futile procedures constitutes not only a betrayal of the donors' trust, but also a frustration for researchers worldwide, who lament the shortage of donor eggs as limiting their research.[19]

In addition, Hwang has wasted not only the time of many scientists, commentators and clinicians worldwide, but also his own time. As a man of not inconsiderable technical skill, he could have put his time and skills to a much more productive use, and could have continued to utilise his expertise well into the future. As it is, this has all come to an end.

In science, as in all other areas of life, what we have has been entrusted to us. In scientific research, the money comes from grant-awarding bodies, governments, or private benefactors. In Christian terms, all these sources are ultimately dependent upon God, who has entrusted to us life itself, our abilities, and our resources (1 Chronicles 29:11,14b). For Christians, this is nothing less than a sacred trust, bestowing upon us a sacred duty to deploy wisely and well our time and our opportunities. To squander these is to demean all that we are as God's redeemed people.

Fraud is hypocritical

At the root of fraud lies hypocrisy and pretence. While promoting an image of themselves as exceptionally successful, fraudsters are corrupt; they are the Pharisees of the scientific world. They set out to be first in society at the expense of the welfare and wellbeing of others, using deception to promote themselves and their own interests.

When scientists commit fraud, they pretend to have expertise, skills and data they do not possess. They are little more than actors, passing themselves off as something they are not. (Matthew 23:25–28) Tragically, they give the impression they are the real thing, with

18   S. Chong, Report: 'Hwang received 2221 Oocytes for Stem Cell Research', *Science*NOW, Daily News, 2 February 2006. Available at: http://sciencenow. sciencemag.org/cgi/content/full/2006/202/1?rss=1. Accessed 27 March 2006.
19   Stojkovic et al, 'Derivation of a human blastocyst', 2005.

real results, and indicating new profitable directions. In reality, they are hollow, dragging the scientific enterprise down and demeaning it.

Whenever this spirit enters science, it has lost the core of how it functions. The alignment of science today with economic and national imperatives has the potential to destroy the scientific enterprise. This is far from inevitable, and yet it surfaces all too commonly in current biotechnology. The Hwang debacle is a tragic example.

Whilst it would be unfair to condemn all commercial link-ups between university scientists and spin-off companies, enormous care is always required. Once we enter a world where there is a 'rich list' of academic scientists, we enter a world where the 'love of money' might begin to exercise far too much influence. (1 Timothy 6:9–10) The search for truth and the lure of financial rewards may well be antithetical, and in science the consequences can be devastating for the nature of the scientific enterprise, as well as for the individuals concerned.

Lessons for Theology

Science lives by stringent and unforgiving rules; its ethos is hard and it has little leeway for the mediocre, let alone for the openly fraudulent. The core of science is that experiments have to be capable of being tested and refuted. If they do not lend themselves to this, they are deemed to be poor experiments. While the rash of fraudulent publications is a deep embarrassment to scientists, fraudulent work has a very short lifespan, even if it is not detected. The ideas will wither if they are incapable of being reproduced. True, a scientist may garner glory for a time, but that glory will dim if the work does not lead in significant directions. The glory will be short-lived. Scientific ideas are always open to being ruthlessly tested, even if human prestige and biased assessments limit this for a time.

When there are major frauds in science, the whole of science is damaged. In the case of Hwang, the realm of stem cells and especially embryonic stem cells has been detrimentally affected. While it may recover, it has been tainted for a time. Credibility is crucial to science; without it there is no reason why anyone should take it seriously.

Can the same be said for other disciplines? Can it be said for theology? Is there such a phenomenon as fraud in theology, or in the claims of Christians? Or is this going too far? Perhaps it is more appropriate to ask whether there is bad or deceptive or misleading theology? And if so, what are the criteria one might use to detect it?

How does one recognise a credible theologian? Surely it is not in terms of whether the theologian in question comes to the conclusions that please us, or that conform to our own theological persuasion. There must be objective ways of coming to a judgement, but what are these ways?

We realise that these may be little more than impertinent, and even irrelevant, questions. After all, we write as non-theologians, and intruding into other disciplinary areas can be a hazardous occupation. Fraud may be of peculiar relevance to science, with its data and its observations which can be mishandled and misconstrued (let alone manufactured). But surely there are commonly accepted interpretive principles in theology that are open to being misused or even ignored. The term 'fraud' may be inappropriate, but there must be acceptable and unacceptable approaches within theology.

It is very difficult to believe that some do not manipulate theological approaches for their own benefit and ends (maybe for financial gains and personal power). Even in the early church false prophets and false teachers were rife (1 Timothy 1:3–7, 2 Peter 2), causing division and strife within the churches. Theology is not immune from the plague of deception, and even fraud, which is causing such havoc in the scientific community. A lack of integrity, honesty, humility and openness to the contribution of others besmirches every human activity, penetrating even into the heart of the church.

Using some of the issues that have emerged in connection with scientific fraud, we can explore this realm in a little more detail.

While theologians might not have commercial link-ups with companies, they may well develop close liaisons with governments. Instead of having a prophetic edge, they may align themselves with dominant political philosophies. In this way, they may expect to attain and wield moral power in the political sphere. The dangers of such liaisons are easy to see, as the distinction between political influence and religious persuasion blurs.

Excessive claims in the theological sphere are little different from overblown claims in the scientific realm. Consider claims for physical healing. One has to question whether 'cures' emanating from the Christian faith healer are any different from the prospects held out by clinicians touting the latest wonder drug. In both cases, the claims have to be backed up by reliable, honest evidence, and both should be approached with a healthy degree of scepticism. Then again, there are the cult leaders, whose authority stems from messianic-style claims based on spurious interpretation of scripture. Underlying deception of this order is a serious re-direction of biblical teaching onto oneself rather than onto Jesus as Lord. Such deception also leads to those situations where members tithe to provide the 'pastor' or leader with a sumptuous lifestyle, in conspicuous contrast to that of ordinary members. The similarities between instances like these and the Hwang affair are striking, characterised as they all are by deception and fraud.

The tragedy of theological deception is that people are led astray, lives are ruined and hopes are dashed. People are disillusioned when confronted by a false gospel rather than the honesty and hope of the true one. The cause of Christianity may be severely dented by poor exegesis of scripture, undue emphasis on charismatic leaders and ecclesiastical chicanery, and an impoverished version of a Christ-like life. Nevertheless, we have to see past these false imitations of the real thing, just as we have to see beyond the scientific fraud and unhelpful short-cuts.

And yet there may be an uneasy difference between theological and scientific fraud, in that the latter may be more readily detected and curbed than might the former. Scientific fraud will be found out, and the ideas based on fraud will ultimately wither. Can the same be said of theological fraud?

From our standpoint as scientists, it is our task to draw these matters to the attention of theologians. It is relatively easy to dismiss science and its worldview when fraud rises to the surface, and fraud has to be tackled by those within the scientific community. However, equally rigorous standards are required of those engaged in allied disciplines, especially theology.

Expecting too much of Science

It is easy to demonise scientists, casting them as single-minded, driven men and women who will happily abandon common morality in their pursuit of scientific breakthroughs and the subsequent prestige. However, they are not alone in wanting to forge ahead into new realms. As human beings we seek to better our world, both personal and communal, and increasingly we turn to science to supply the solutions. Our expectation of what science can do for us has vastly increased as advance after advance has been made. However, these expectations are sometimes too high.

Surprisingly, this discussion overlaps with that which will be conducted in the later chapter on enhancement and transhumanism. The idealistic vistas of the latter raise the hopes of many, as illnesses of all descriptions will be conquered and age itself will be defeated. Such possibilities are usually discussed in the context of whether or not goals of this sort are desirable. And yet there might be an even greater problem. How are these end-points to be reached? The expectations of the general public are being unrealistically raised, but they will inevitably be dashed. Alongside this, are the expectations of some scientists also being unrealistically raised? In their case, rather than have their hopes dashed, will they manipulate results to give the impression that the goals have actually been attained (or, at least, partially so)? The pressures being generated by transhumanists are immense, and will increase yet further if their creed becomes more widespread. What is at present the province of a limited number of enthusiasts could have major consequences for the tenor of biomedical science and its thinking.

Scientists function within a cultural context, responding to the hopes and expectations of their society and its members. It only takes a minority of scientists influenced by excessive commercial interest or idealistic transhumanist perspectives to take a fraudulent path, and the reputation of science is tarnished.

A dispassionate and critical appraisal of scientific claims is always in order. Indeed, such an appraisal is essential for the wellbeing of the whole scientific endeavour. Extravagant claims and media hype are the downfall of science. But exactly the same can be said of theology and Christian claims. Miraculous claims and spiritual hype need to be approached with the same vigilance and careful discernment. Exaggeration and excessive dogmatic certainty can be just as destructive of Christian claims as are overstatements and false assertions within the scientific arena. All are destructive of truth.

It is in this context that we have to view science and the pressures upon it. We should not expect science to be immune to its cultural context. It is not, but neither is theology. By the same token, we should not expect the way in which science is conducted today to be the same as in the 1950s. Its results and technological offshoots will be used by some to push moral boundaries in ways others will not approve of. But that is the world in which we find ourselves.

D. GARETH JONES

The Human Body:
An Anatomist's Journey from Death to Life

Introduction

Of all the subject areas within bioethics, the one that tends to be most neglected is the way in which we are to treat the dead human body. Exactly the same applies to theological thinking, which seems to have had little to say about the dead body. However, for many centuries there has been widespread belief that dissection of the human body is an act of desecration; a belief prevalent even today in some circles, including certain Christian ones.

In mediaeval times the Roman Catholic church and popes had to interact with anatomists who sought to dissect bodies of the recently deceased. To take one example, Pope Clement VI (1291–1352) mandated autopsies of victims of bubonic plague.[1] A short time earlier, Pope Boniface VIII had declared that whoever cut up a body or boiled it would fall under the church's ban.[2] Nevertheless, it is not thought that this was directed at prohibiting dissection in medical schools.

In theological thinking today, one comes across considerable debate on the body in its various manifestations: the spiritual or resurrection body over against the natural or mortal body; the relationship between body, soul and spirit; and the ways in which humans and their bodies image God, their creator. Important as are all such

---

1   C. B. Rodning, "'O death, where is thy sting?" Historical perspectives on the relationship of human postmortem anatomical dissection to medical education and care', *Clinical Anatomy* 2, 1989, pp.277–92.

2   K. Park, 'The life of the corpse: Division and dissection in late Medieval Europe', *Journal of the History of Medicine and Allied Sciences* 50, 1995, pp.111–32.

discussions, they are far removed from providing clues as to how we think about the bodily remains of those who have died. One gains the impression that this topic is of very little interest to contemporary Christians; it may even be considered irrelevant. But this has not always been the case.

There was a time when considerable store was placed not only on burial of the body, but burial in consecrated ground. This was seen as a fit resting place for the mortal remains of a once living person, a reminder of what that person was in life, and very often a reminder of the pain and anguish they had had to bear. Not only did this provide a clear recognition of the connection between the person who once lived and that person's dead body, but also between the person who walked among us and that person now in heaven.

Considerations such as these are of limited value, however, in providing tools with which to answer questions about what can or cannot be done to dead bodies, or what relationship there should be between the wishes of the now deceased regarding what is to be done to their body at death and the feelings of living relatives. Neither do they throw light on the myriad issues surrounding the donation of organs harvested from cadavers.

Emerging Attitudes towards the Human Body

Three to four hundred years ago in Europe there was intense interest in the interior of the human body, that which lay beneath the skin and muscles. This hidden territory intrigued people, and not simply the thinkers and philosophers of the day. Popular culture, the mass media of the time, was unable to escape its perplexing and fascinating mysteries. What was the heart like, or the liver or the gut? Without X-rays, let alone CT (computer-assisted tomography) scans or MRI (magnetic resonance imaging), this was a mysterious and even superstitious world. Its hiddenness was perplexing.

It was onto this dark and threatening territory that dissection began to shed some light. And yet this was far from straightforward, since the dissection of dead bodies was hardly commonly accepted practice. After all, bodies were not routinely available for dissection, and the ones that did become available came directly from the gallows. And, on top of this, the anatomy theatres were places where professor-centred performances took place. Not surprisingly, every aspect of the process was designed to elicit morbid curiosity. Nothing could have been further from today's sanitised, scientific environment.

The criminals whose bodies were undergoing dissection, the executioners responsible for making the bodies available, and the anatomists whose profession depended upon this supply of bodies, were united in 'the culture of dissection'. All were involved in an orchestrated series of events taking place on the edges of respectable society, barely accepted, dubious and perhaps even taboo. Unsurprisingly, the act of dissecting the bodies of criminals was talked about in the language of treason, treachery, duplicity and secrecy.[3]

Even more difficult for us today are the accounts given by some of the poets and writers of the time, as they outlined their dreams of dissection. But stranger still are the erotic verses in which poets expressed their desires for their loved ones by describing in intimate detail their dissection. To some of these seventeenth-century poets, this was the ultimate in physical surrender. Listen to Richard Lovelace's 1659 poem in which he addresses his mistress:

> Ah my fair Murdresse! Dost thou cruelly heal,
> With Various pains to make me well?
> Then let me be
> Thy cut Anatomie
> And in each mangled part my heart you'l see.

In spite of their being active participants in the execution process,[4] anatomists at this time were viewed surprisingly well by society, their involvement being recognised as having a divine quality. This was because the dissected shell of the body provided a medium with which

3   J. Sawday, *The Body Emblazoned* (London: Routledge, 1995).
4   R. Richardson, *Death, Dissection and the Destitute* (London: Penguin Books, 1988).

to understand the creative intent of God.[5] Consequently, the interior of the body was viewed as a sacred temple, and not simply the remains of a once living person.

One of the cultural devices used at that time was the genre of self-dissection. In this, the dead body is depicted as being an accomplice in the process of dissection, apparently having carried out the dissection itself. Many examples are found in the art of the period, where the onlooker is left wondering whether the dissected body (standing and sometime provocatively posed) is alive or dead. Who is doing the dissection: is it the anatomist or the cadaver? Strange as this question might seem, the impresssion was given that knowledge of the dead body was actually knowledge of the living. What this did was to stress the naturalness of dissection.

Along these same lines, dissected cadavers were sometimes portrayed as existing on the fringes of living society. It was as if they constituted a new community of the dead. In depicting cadavers in this way, anatomists such as Vesalius and their illustrators were providing a commentary on human destiny, as much as on human structure. They appear to be saying that the anatomist was not disrupting the body so much as the body was willingly allowing the anatomist to assist the general process of decay and dissolution. This was an important justification for the practice of anatomy and dissection.[6]

Strange as these ideas seem to us, they convey a message of considerable contemporary potency: that anatomy and dissection can never be self-justifying regimes.[7] They always exist in cultural contexts that either accept or reject procedures such as these. They must always be justified, because they always transcend normal ethical boundaries. These considerations are also important within a Christian perspective, where the integrity of the body is generally cherished and upheld. Can anatomical investigations of the human body ever be justified, and, if so, on what grounds?

5   D. G. Jones, *Speaking for the Dead* (Aldershot: Ashgate, 2000).
6   Sawday, *The Body Emblazoned.*
7   Jones, *Speaking for the Dead.*

A Modern Eruption

The lack of serious thinking about the ethical issues surrounding the use of the human body and human remains has left anatomists and many other medical people peculiarly unprepared to meet the new challenges of very recent years. This is due in no small measure to the advent of 'plastination', with the emergence of what has become known as 'anatomy art'.[8] This is based on an exhibition, *Body Worlds*, which is directed at the general public. Instead of being largely hidden from public view in dissecting rooms and museums, cadavers are now on general display in large exhibition spaces, surrounded by fanfares of publicity and ardent debate.

The dead bodies are prepared through the process of plastination, in which human tissues are impregnated with plastics and silicone rubber. The resulting specimens are permanent, and are also dry and odourless. Additionally, tissues can be moulded, enabling body parts to be fixed in various positions.

In the hands of those with artistic skills, the end result is a display of human bodies exhibiting postures of walking, running, and sitting. In turn, these figures can be used to illustrate basic anatomical and physiological functions. The organisation of body systems such as the digestive, respiratory and urinary systems can be demonstrated in appropriately dissected body regions. Cross-sections of the body can be used to display bones, muscles, organs and vessels in amazing detail: precise and accurate.

As if this were not sufficient, the exhibits need not be confined to healthy bodies; the effects of disease processes can be readily demonstrated and explained. What are the effects of smoking on lungs, or of alcohol on the liver? What do artificial joints, such as hips or knees, look like?

Using these procedures, dead human bodies give the appearance of being very lifelike plastic models of the human body. The shock is to realise that these are not models but real (dead) people, who were

8   G. Von Hagens, *Anatomy Art*, Catalogue on the exhibition (Heidelberg: Institute of Plastination, 2000).

once living and breathing and thinking, just like us. Instead of having been buried or cremated, there they are standing before us, albeit in a dissected state. It is this very lifelikeness that both attracts and appals the onlooker.

This begins to explain what all the fuss is about. This is a new way of depicting and demonstrating the dead human body. In some quarters, these entities are now being called 'plastinates',[9] though whether this helps or hinders an understanding of what they really are is a question for debate. Although plastination is used extensively in academic anatomy departments for teaching and research purposes, whole bodies are not displayed in such dramatic fashion. There is no need to do so for teaching at university level: all that is required in a medical school is plastination to demonstrate the structure of organs, or the relationship between muscles, nerves and vessels in the limbs, trunk, and head and neck.

This is anatomy with a far more public facade than it has had for 200 years. City after city, in country after country, has been exposed to this form of modern anatomy with its very disconcerting context. The *Body Worlds* exhibition has been held in recent years in countries as diverse as Belgium and Japan, Austria and Taiwan. Cities to have hosted it include London, Houston, Toronto, Seoul and Singapore.

These issues are profound ones, since these uses of plastinated human bodies are innovative and disconcerting. They also force the general public to confront their own responses to the dead human body. This use of plastination carries us a very long way indeed from traditional anatomy and probably from traditional ways of treating the human body. What can or should be done to dead human bodies? Are these uses transgressing important boundaries, and do they by their very nature demean our humanity? Is human dignity at stake?

9   See: http://www.bodyworlds.com/en/pages/home.asp.

Challenging Ethical Issues

Central to the ethical debate is whether the people, when they were alive, bequeathed their bodies to be used in this manner.[10] Did they give fully informed consent, and did they give it freely? While informed consent by itself is not sufficient to justify exhibitions of this type, it is the crucial underlying prerequisite.[11] The organisers of the *Body Worlds* exhibitions are adamant that they have obtained such consent, and a detailed information booklet, 'Donating your body for plastination', is produced by the Institute for Plastination, Heidelberg, and is available on their website.[12]

The crucial question to be asked is what is the nature of these exhibitions? For some, they are solely educational in nature, although others recognise in them an artistic element. In all probability they are a mixture of the two. But to what extent are they entertainment, in the sense that their organisers have set out principally to entertain those who attend? Of course, since death is on display, it may be impossible to escape from some voyeuristic overtones.

These considerations are not merely theoretical, and apply not only to the public exhibitions. After all, many researchers use human bodies and tissues in their studies, and all are heavily dependent upon public sentiment condoning such activities. Without that support, any use of the human body could be regarded as an affront to human dignity.

Society condones a range of uses of dead human bodies and body parts. These include dissection, autopsies, the retention of human parts and organs for further investigations, the use of some of this material in museums, as well as research on human material. Appropriate consent has been given in each case and for approved uses. In most instances the justification stems from an educational, scientific or clinical rationale. The stipulations are needed, since all human tissue

10   D. G. Jones, 'Use of bequeathed and unclaimed bodies in the dissecting room', *Clinical Anatomy* 7, 1994, pp.102–107.
11   D. G. Jones, *Clinical Anatomy* 20, 2007, pp.338–43.
12   For the web address see footnote 9.

is an object of moral interest, coming as it does from one or more members of the human community.

This is the ethical and cultural context within which all exhibitions have to be assessed. Do they have a museum ethos or have they toppled over into the realm of peep-shows? Are the bodies of real people being used to titillate and allure rather than teach something substantial about the human body? The boundary is a tentative one, as it always is when dealing with cadavers. Plastination makes it far easier to convert serious education into fickle entertainment, and even to confuse the two.[13]

As an anatomist, I contend that, with appropriate ethical constraints, it is ethically legitimate to make use of the human body and body parts to help understand the body and its workings. On the other hand, its use for purely artistic ends, where the goal is to employ actual human material to enhance works of art, takes us into different territory. This is a world far removed from the anatomical studies and sketches of Leonardo da Vinci (1452–1519) and Andreas Vesalius (1514–1564). Revolutionary as their work then was, it *depicted* the dissected human body rather than *incorporated* it into their work. In doing this, it accomplished both artistic and educational ends.

At the other extreme are more recent notorious examples of unethical activities: the incorporation of human foetuses in jewellery and human material in sculptures. The artists could have achieved their purposes without the use of actual human material that, as a result, was being employed exclusively to serve the interests of the artist. They teach us nothing about the human body or human tissue; in fact, the objects may actually cause moral harm since human interests are being demeaned and exploited.[14]

Where do exhibitions such as *Body Worlds* fit in? At a general level, one might argue that we have to balance the extent to which public displays of plastinated human bodies are capable of enhancing people's understanding of the structure and function of the human body, against the extent to which they are being used for voyeuristic

---

13   D. G. Jones, 'The use of human tissue: An insider's view', *New Zealand Bioethics Journal* 3(2), 2002, pp.8–12.
14   Jones, *Speaking for the Dead.*

or artistic ends. Inevitably, different visitors to these exhibitions will find themselves at different points along this continuum, but this applies to any visit to any conventional museum.

Elements of a Christian Response

But is this adequate? Is this as far as we can go, and are there no helpful insights to be obtained from the Christian church? Might a Christian perspective assist in our response? Alternatively, it may be that there is no Christian perspective, and that Christians have no contribution to make.

Whenever approached by the media, church spokespeople tend to object to shows of this nature and, sometimes, even call for them to be banned. The reasons for this reaction are likely to be on the grounds that the body is sacred, and that they are dishonouring the body, or that the dignity of human beings is being compromised. The assertion is sometimes made that a moral and ethical line is being crossed, with displays of bodies amounting to a desecration of all we hold dear. The question we have to face is whether such a reactionary response emanates from a considered theological base, or whether it is super-ficial and unhelpful.

Before exploring these issues in more detail, what clues do we get as to the views of the biblical writers on the dead human body? A first element stems from examples in both Old and New Testaments of the high view held of the dead body. An example of this is found in Amos, who specifically separates out for condemnation the crimes of one group of people who, not content with marauding, pillaging and killing, unleashed their venom on the body of one of their enemies. Having killed the king of Edom (Amos 2:1–3), they burnt his bones to ash. Not content with killing him, they then desecrated his dead body, thereby undermining his integrity as an individual.[15]

---

15   D. G. Jones, 'The human cadaver: An assessment of the value we place on the dead body', *Perspectives on Science and Christian Faith* 47, 1995, pp.43–51.

Another instance of the significance ascribed to the dead body is provided by Joseph who, prior to his death, had his relatives promise to take his bones with them to the land of Canaan when they were finally able to leave Egypt. (Genesis 50:22–26, Exodus 13:19) Dead though he would be, Joseph did not want his mortal remains to be left in Egypt, the land of captivity. This may have been symbolic, and yet it strengthens the notion that the dead body is sufficiently important to require commitment on the part of others. In the New Testament, we find that, following Jesus' death, his followers carefully and sacrificially tended his body. (Matthew 27:57–61, Mark 15:42–16, Luke 23:50–24, John 19:38–42) They considered it inappropriate to leave his body on the cross, especially as this would have meant leaving it there over the sabbath day. Joseph of Arimathea ensured that Jesus' body was laid in his own new tomb, while a number of his followers, among them Nicodemus and Mary Magdalene, were concerned that the body was anointed with spices and bound according to Jewish custom. While there are many cultural factors coming into play here, there is no hint that Jesus disapproved of their actions. There was nothing untoward in looking after his dead body in this way. His followers may have underestimated the likelihood of his resurrection, but that was another matter. What is encountered in these instances is a clear recognition that the dead body is something to be treated with respect.

This conclusion is not in any way surprising, since there is no suggestion in the Bible that human beings can have any existence apart from the body, even in the future life after death. In unequivocal terms, Paul enunciated the point that the resurrection is a physical one (1 Corinthians 15:42–52, 1 Thessalonians 4:13–18), a belief foreshadowed in the Old Testament. (Daniel 12:2) A biblical view, therefore, militates against any idea of humans existing apart from some bodily manifestation or form of expression.[16] The mortal body we now know will be replaced by a resurrection body, a form of spiritual body, which while not identical to our present material body has sufficient similarities to it to warrant the term 'body'. Jesus' own resurrection

16   B. O. Banwell, *The Illustrated Bible Dictionary* (Leicester: Inter-Varsity Press, 1980), pp.202–203.

body serves as the only guide we have to this (Luke 24:12,31), with its recognisably human and personal features but also its ability to pass through material objects and leave no corpse.

Bearing this similarity in mind, we can go further and argue that respect for the dead body *now* foreshadows respect for the resurrection body *in the future*. While in no way suggesting that there is a close parallel between the two, there would appear to be connections. A willingness to desecrate or devalue the dead body shows a disregard for what that person might become, as much as it shows a disregard for what that person has been. While it is not our prerogative to judge what any person might be like in eternity, it is our responsibility to provide support and protection as far as we know how. A Christian perspective, therefore, has to have regard to this future dimension in determining how a dead body is to be treated in the present, taking account of the notion that this present life is preparation for a future one. An element within this perspective is that the prior wishes of the deceased are respected as far as possible, since our bodies constitute the one common strand between what we are now and what we may become.

Hence, while a Christian response might have similarities to many general ethical stances, it goes further by recognising that the dead body serves as a link between what that person has been and what that person may become. It imparts a future orientation to add to the past orientation of general ethical perspectives. The body itself is an inadequate token of these dimensions, but it is all that remains. It is a reminder of the greater ongoing dimensions of human existence, and also of the reality of our limitations and needs, as well as of our mortality. We shall all die and be like this one before us, who is now dead. Respect for the dead body reminds us, not only of the significance of the one who has died, but of the significance of all human life. Consequently, to value the dead body is to value the person, and to see that person as one who mirrors God. To devalue the dead body is to devalue those still alive, and also to call into question the purposes and intentions of God in creating people in his image.

But what amounts to devaluing the dead person? Does plastination inevitably do this? What about far better known examples such as dissection, along with organ transplantation and donation? Perhaps those church spokespeople were right all along: we should oppose any public display of bodies. Or were they?

The Role of Informed Consent and Altruism

There can be no doubt that dissection amounts to mutilation of the body; perhaps it is the ultimate in desecration of the body? I shall argue that the latter does not follow from the former: mutilation does not inevitably lead to desecration. One crucial factor prevents this, and this is the role played by informed consent.[17,18] It is this that transforms what would otherwise be an act of desecration into an act of respect, simply because what is then done with and to the body is a fulfilment of the considered wishes of the person when still alive. Undergirding these wishes is the person's altruism, the gifting of their dead body to others. The aim is to ensure that their body is put to good use, namely, education and/or research, so that people in future will benefit from this gift. Their life has come to an end, but their mortal remains may be able to assist others in some way.

This is a crucial perspective both ethically and theologically, since it enables the dead body to be put to uses which would not otherwise be permissible. The only way in which this perspective of respect and a dissection ethos can be held together is via altruism.[19] In these terms, the sole justification for dissection within a Christian perspective stems from the altruism of the living, in that the person when alive decided to gift their body to a medical school in order to be used in a certain way following death. The specific Christian thrust

17   Retained Organs Commission, *A Consultation Document on Unclaimed and Unidentified Organs and Tissue: A Possible Regulatory Framework*, (National Health Service, London, 2002).

18   Department of Health, *The Removal, Retention and Use of Human Organs and Tissue from Postmortem Examination*, (Her Majesty's Stationery Office, London, 2001).

19   W. F. May, 'Religious justification for donating body parts', *Hastings Center Report* 15, 1985, pp.38–42.

within this principle is that the supreme model available is that of Jesus himself, in giving up his own life for others. To give one's life for one's friends is ethically commendable, but to do it for those who are undeserving is the height of altruism. (John 15:13) In becoming a human being, and then in giving up that life voluntarily for others, Jesus demonstrated in unequivocal terms the characteristics of a life of humility rather than of arrogance or conceit. (Philippians 2:3–8) The gift of one's body after death in no way matches altruism of this calibre; it is, therefore, a limited form of altruism. Nevertheless, it is imbued with the essence of altruism.

In the light of this, it is easy to appreciate that the same applies to the donation of organs for transplantation. In this case, one might argue that the thrust is an even more powerful one, since the aim is to save the life of someone else, or to prolong a life debilitated by disease. The organ of someone now dead is being employed to enrich the life of someone still alive.[20] I am giving something for which I no longer have any use to someone who is desperately in need of what I can give. Once again the central ethical and theological driving force is that this is done willingly, seeking the good of someone else rather than my own good. Neither I, nor my close family, get anything in return; it is a charitable act; it is one of love. By acting in this way, people make a gift of something more closely identified than anything else with what they are and represent.

The thrust of altruism is that the giving of one's body is to be preferred to coercion; giving is better than taking, and the good of others is better than self-interest. In line with this principle, bequests are preferable to the use of unclaimed bodies, while an opt-in scheme for organ donation is preferable to an opt-out scheme. The latter has limited ethical merit, since it lacks an altruistic element. Something (a body or organ) is taken without permission, the person from whom it is taken having no means of defending their own bodily integrity.

A further principle stems from the response of many who see death, especially premature or unexpected death, as evil or tragic. Such people may find solace and meaning in the use of body parts to

20   T. H. Murray, 'Gifts of the body and the needs of strangers', *Hastings Center Report* 17, 1987, pp.30–38.

assist others. This is what is sometimes referred to as the 'redemptive aspect' of body or organ donations.[21] The death of one person can be interpreted as conferring life on another. Out of the evil of a tragedy can come new life and hope. Such a transformation of the situation can only occur, however, if the body is willingly donated to a medical school, or if organs are freely given to another in need of them. Consequently, this principle is intimately linked to the autonomy of the donor and to the altruism that donation signifies.[22]

The redemptive aspect underlines the principle that death can be used to bring life to others. An evil can be put to good uses. This is especially so when the death is of a young person and if it has been brought about by evil actions such as those of a drunk driver. This theme is repeated endlessly throughout medical practice, where efforts are devoted towards extracting as much good as possible from evil situations brought about by rampant disease.

Public Displays of Plastinates and Altruism

But where does the public display of plastinated bodies and body parts fit into this scheme of things? Informed consent is as crucial as ever, but is altruism as strong? And what about the redemptive aspects of the donation? Is the body being given to others for good purposes?

The closest parallel is that of dissection, where bodies are dissected for educational reasons. As we have seen, altruism is prominent here, and society benefits from the donations as a result of the education of health science students, and also from research conducted on some of the bodies. But what benefits emerge from the public displays of these so-called plastinates? Firstly, there may well be an educational benefit, with those benefiting on this occasion being

---

21   De Vawter et al., *The Use of Human Fetal Tissue: Scientific, Ethical and Policy Concerns* (Minnesota: University of Minnesota, 1990).
22   Jones, 'The human cadaver'.

the general public. In so far as this is the case, the thrust of altruism is as great here as in dissection.

A second possible benefit is to the world of art. The value of the artistic side to these exhibitions has been advocated in the case of the *Body Worlds* exhibitions, although this has never been totally separated from anatomy, with its focus on increasing understanding of the structure of the human body. It is this 'anatomy art' emphasis that links these plastinates most closely with the great artists and anatomists of the Renaissance period. However, is this benefit worthy of the motive of altruism, or is it a superficial outcome? It is perhaps inappropriate for a scientist to answer this question, but theologically one has to grapple with it. Clearly art is of importance and should be celebrated, but is the price being paid in this instance too high? I shall leave it as a question.

A third benefit to be considered is that of entertainment, since this is undoubtedly a significant side to these exhibitions. Whilst I have been ambivalent with regard to the artistic side, I cannot justify entertainment as being a sufficient rationale for altruism. Even where the donors, when still alive, have given fully informed consent, in that they have known precisely how their bodies will be displayed, this does not justify *any* use of dead bodies. Displaying dead bodies as mere entertainment is degrading, since it demeans all that those bodies have stood for as integral facets of human persons capable of relating to each other and to God.

In practice, of course, there is undoubtedly a mixture of these three possible benefits, with each of education, art and entertainment jostling for pride of place. The ratio of the one to the others is what has to be assessed before one is able to make a reasoned ethical and theological judgement. My conclusion is that, for any such display to be at all justifiable on the grounds of altruism, greatest emphasis has to be placed upon its educational benefit, with a lesser emphasis upon art, and with the entertainment side being of limited consequence.

And yet a nagging concern runs through this whole debate. Does plastination convert cadavers into objects or things in a way that is ethically objectionable? Even accepting that fully informed consent has been given, does plastination objectify bodies in a way not characteristic of any other post-death procedure? Wetz has argued against this notion, on the ground that a cadaver is already an object or thing. He writes:

> It becomes a thing before it comes under the hands of the plastinator. Consequently, the object principle can only relate to living persons, not to dead bodies, as these no longer have a subject quality.[23]

He sees no difference between plastination and the removal of organs or tissues for transplantation or anatomical purposes.

Do Plastinates challenge our Worldview?

But is there still one more consideration that I have ignored up to this juncture? Is there a worldview creeping through these exhibitions that is antagonistic to Christian thinking? Why are these plastinates made to appear as though they are alive? Why are they depicted as though they are living in the same way that you and I are living; sitting, running, playing chess, riding a horse, swimming? What is this saying?

These depictions remind us of the mediaeval sketches of dissected cadavers living on the edge of society, or giving the impression that they had carried out the dissections on themselves.[24] The cadavers were given the appearance of being alive, as though they were a population of the living dead. These exhibitions are doing the same, but within a completely different cultural setting. There is no need any longer to justify anatomy and the dissection of cadavers, as there was a few hundred years ago. And so the motive now must be different. What is it?

My conclusion is that, in the eyes of some, it may be an attempt to escape from the reality of death, by giving the impression that these cadavers are continuing to exist in much the same way as when they were alive. Of course, there are major differences; they are dissected

23   F. J. Wetz, 'The dignity of man', in Von Hagens, *Anatomy Art*, pp. 239–58.
24   Sawday, *The Body Emblazoned*.

in a host of different ways, and yet there is a hint that we can live on as plastinates. This is not the ageless existence that transfixes transhumanists, but plastinates appear to have attained their own form of everlasting existence. Perhaps they have; and yet it is a very impoverished form of everlasting life.

Even this everlasting existence brings with it demanding ethical and theological questions. At some point, decisions will have to be made about how to dispose of this imperishable material that is human and yet not quite human. And is this the point we are searching for? In acquiring some form of everlasting existence have these plastinates ceased to be human? One observer responded in these words:

> Each of ... [the] corpses is, at one level, a perfect human specimen that is a real privilege to observe at close quarters. And yet, the absence of a personality, friends, family and history leaves a gaping and eerie vacuum that forcefully calls into question what it is to be human and reminds us of what few of us like to dwell on – our mortality. They are bodies with no soul.[25]

Everlasting existence may, in one sense, have been achieved, but only by sacrificing the human core. The replacement of dead human tissue with plastics leaves nothing more than plasticised remnants of what was once human, fascinating and yet perplexing, uplifting yet troublesome. We seem to have created a new form of existence, perhaps 'plastinate' is indeed an appropriate term, and yet we have not come to terms with what this means.

It is here that we begin to glimpse the connections between ongoing existence as a plastic remnant of a human, and the transhumanists' vision of an ongoing existence as an apparently ageless, potentially disease-free remnant of a human. While we have little idea whether the latter will ever eventuate, we can sceptically surmise that there will be a vast gulf between a fully functional 30- or 50-year-old and a 150-year-old human 'form'. If the fully functional element is missing, we can ask whether the 150-year-old will be as different from a plastinate as is generally assumed. Both forms of existence might be fitting topics for further theological exploration.

25   E. H. Nicholls, 'Selling anatomy: the role of the soul', *Endeavour* 26(2), 2002, p.47.

D. GARETH JONES

Enhancement: Is Baseless Speculation Misleading Theologians and Bioethicists?

Introduction

While a few commentators argue that we have a moral obligation to enhance human beings, most draw a sharp distinction between therapy and enhancement. *Therapeutic* procedures aimed at restoring individuals to normality are generally applauded, whereas *enhancement* procedures, those aimed at improving individuals by providing them with abilities they would not otherwise have possessed, are usually decried. This distinction gives the impression of being straightforward, and yet it is based on questionable premises, namely, that the boundaries of normality are self-evident and static and that all forms of enhancement are unacceptable.

A World of Enhancement Fantasies

It is not unusual to encounter stories in serious newspapers and magazines with headlines such as 'Anyone for tennis, at the age of 150?' or 'Do you want to live to be 800?' Aubrey de Grey, a biogerontologist at Cambridge University, argues that a future world, perhaps 1,000 years hence, could be populated with people who are alive today and are already around 60 years of age. According to this scenario, the concept of ageing will have become obsolete, with a world populated by people enjoying a state of eternal youth, and no longer threatened by the major diseases of the twenty-first century.[1]

Along similar lines, Ronald Bailey envisages a typical family reunion at the end of the present century. At this reunion there are five generations gathered together, with the oldest member, at 150, playing tennis with her 30-year-old great-great-granddaughter.[2] On the eve of the twenty-second century, diabetes, Parkinson's disease and AIDS will have been consigned to the past, tissues and organs will be readily regenerated, and human immortality will beckon. Technologies using stem cells, constructing artificial chromosomes and creating perfect transplants will together have transformed our vision of human nature.

My use of the term 'fantasies' in the section heading is not meant to deride the possibilities contained within these depictions. Rather, it is to denote the tenor of so much of the debate within the enhancement domain. Fantasies and what appear to be far-flung visions sit alongside one another.

Such visions are being worked out in some detail by one author after another. For instance, Joel Garreau[3] writes:

> We are at a turning point in history. For millenniums our technologies ... have been aimed at modifying our environment. Now, for the first time, our technologies are increasingly aimed inward – at altering our minds, memories, metabolisms, personalities, and progeny. This is not some science fiction future. Inexorable increases in ingenuity are opening vistas, especially in what we may call GRIN – genetic, robotic, information and nano-technologies.[4]

What is science fiction and what is science fact? Is such thinking as this nothing more than scientistic hyperbole, or are we obligated to overcoming limitations imposed upon us by our genes and our environment? However we react to possibilities of this sort, we are at

1   B. McCall, 'Do you want to live to be 800? This man says that you can', *The Times Higher Education Supplement*, 10 March 2006.
2   R. Bailey, 'Anyone for tennis, at the age of 150', *The Times*, 8 April 2006.
3   J. Garreau, *Radical Evolution: The Promise and Peril of Enhancing our Minds, our Bodies – and What it Means to be Human*, (New York: Doubleday, 2005).
4   J. Garreau, 'Let humanity prevail', *The Times Higher Education Supplement*, 11 August 2005.

once confronted by profound philosophical, ethical and theological conundrums.

One philosopher who deals with some of these issues is Jürgen Habermas. In his book *The Future of Human Nature*, he expresses considerable concern at the prospects opened up by enhancement, against the background of the presumed efficiency of genetic intervention. He writes:

> Eugenic interventions aiming at enhancement, reduce ethical freedom insofar as they tie down the person concerned to rejected, but irreversible intentions of third parties, barring him from the spontaneous self-perception of being the undivided author of his own life.[5]

In view of this he argues that:

> The programmed person ... may feel the lack of a mental precondition for coping with the moral expectation to take, even if only in retrospect, the *sole* responsibility for her own life.[6]

Although Habermas's primary concern is with genetic programming, he views pre-implantation genetic diagnosis (PGD) as being tarred with the same perfectionist brush. With this in mind he views PGD selection as being:

> based on a judgment of the quality of a human being and therefore express[ing] a desire for genetic optimisation. An act that in the end leads to the selection of a healthier organism issues from the same attitude as a eugenic praxis.[7]

Underlying positions like these is the assumption that there is a very close relationship between futuristic visions of medical accomplishments and present reality. Running through all these grandiose visions of human self-modification, genetic perfectibility, and eugenic aspirations, is the notion of biological enhancement. Furthermore, the boundaries between these visions and current medical practice have been obliterated.

5   J Habermas, *The Future of Human Nature* (Cambridge: Polity Press, 2003).
6   Ibid., pp.81, 82.
7   Ibid., p.97.

Theological Opposition to Enhancement

In the light of these viewpoints, we need to ask whether there are any theological perspectives that might prove of assistance. At first sight it appears that, generally speaking, the theological perspectives on offer are reactionary, responding to extreme scenarios represented by trans-humanism (to which I shall later return) rather than assessing what enhancement actually entails.

Cameron is forthright in dismissing any hint of enhancement in the form of 'better babies' or 'super-health'.[8] He sees fundamental problems in many instances where there is technological intrusion into human life, which he views as redesigning what we are as humans. And so he envisions that, when Jesus returns, instead of finding fellow members of *Homo sapiens*, he will find self-invented, designer beings. The message, I imagine, is that followers of Christ ought to shun any whiff of any technology even remotely associated with enhancement possibilities.

A central theme picked up by some Christian writers is that enhancement represents perfection through technology.[9] This is some-times referred to as the Baconian project, according to which modern biomedical technology is driven by a desire to relieve human subjection to fate or necessity.[10] Emphasis is placed on the power of this form of technology, the goal of which is seen as overcoming the vulnerability of the human body.[11] If taken far enough, this might amount to nothing less than a redefinition of human traits and con-ditions. And so, it is argued, if God is no longer considered the author

---

8   N. de S. Cameron, 'The pursuit of enhancement', *Christianity Today*, 22 Feb-ruary 2006; http://www.christianitytoday.com/ct/2006/108/32.0.html.

9   C. Deane-Drummond, 'Future Perfect? God, the transhuman future and the quest for immortality', in *Future Perfect?* (London: T. and T. Clark Inter-national, 2006), pp.168–82.

10   G. McKenny, *To Relieve the Human Condition: Bioethics, Technology, and the Body* (Albany: State University of New York Press, 1997).

11   G. McKenny, 'Enhancements and the ethical significance of vulnerability', in *Enhancing Human Traits: Ethical and Social Implications*, ed. E. Parens (Washington DC: Georgetown University Press, 1998).

of nature, the use of enhancement technologies opens the way for human beings to reconstruct their bodies and brains in the absence of any moral or theological framework.

Hence, Celia Deane-Drummond is concerned that 'a mortality-denying, imperfection-denying culture will not be able to accept mortality and imperfection ...'[12] Consequently, efforts might well be directed towards utilising biological means to bring about bodily perfection, and an ageless, disease-free bodily existence. From a theological perspective, this is a radical misunderstanding of the notion of perfection, which has always focused on the development of character and human virtues, even where there is bodily imperfection and frequently in the face of substantial flaws in the body. Perfection has been seen as belonging to God and as stemming from God, and ultimately as being unattainable in this life and in this body. Its future-orientation and God-centredness have gone together.

Junker-Kenny[13] is equally concerned with what she regards as this thrust towards self-perfection and biological sources of perfectibility. She considers that help is not to be found in any genetic enhancement but in knowing oneself and one's limits. She argues that, instead of defining ourselves through acquiring optimal genes, we should be looking to the human capacity for finding fulfilment in the face of genetic and other obstacles. Her concern is that, by enhancing performance, we may destroy the source of competence, and we may transform something unique into something typical. She wants us to re-imagine perfection by placing emphasis upon a person's God-consciousness and, therefore, upon traits such as being merciful. This stands in radical opposition to any attempts at achieving perfection through genetic means.

In critiquing enhancement technologies as means of achieving perfection, theologians such as these are alarmed at efforts to attain a

---

12   C. E. Deane-Drummond, 'How might a virtue ethic frame debates in human genetics?', in *Brave New World? Theology, Ethics, and the Human Genome*, ed. C. E. Deane-Drummond (London: T. and T. Clark International, 2003), pp. 225–52, p.235.

13   M. Junker-Kenny, 'Genetic perfection, or fulfilment of creation in Christ?', in *Future Perfect?* (London: T. and T. Clark International, 2006), pp.155–67.

state of 'better than well'[14] or 'better than human'.[15] Their critique of medical efforts at enhancement amounts to nothing less than a critique of using the medical enterprise to transform humans into posthumans. It appears that they think of enhancement as a religious enterprise diametrically opposed to Christian aspirations. In their view, concepts such as finitude, perfection and immortality are being reinterpreted, divesting them of any God-centred identity.

But are these critiques being fair to the many medical procedures that may have only some overtones of enhancement? Or are they over-reactions to an extreme version of enhancement, and are they thereby unhelpful or even misleading? This is an issue to which I shall return later.

Brent Waters identifies two possible responses to these more extreme possibilities: to view humans as co-creators who use technology and medicine to work with God in constructing a new creation, or to use theology as a counter discourse.[16] Waters opts for the latter, arguing that technology is not to be used by human beings to eliminate either the finite or the mortal limits that define humans as embodied creatures. In other words, he takes as his starting point these extreme scenarios. Some theologians, however, work within a less catastrophic framework, acknowledging that human beings are indeed called to develop themselves, with the result that some enhancement of their capacities may be appropriate and even required.[17]

An ostensibly non-theological critique, but with clear theological concerns, is that contained in the report of the President's Council on Bioethics.[18] The essential sources of concern that emanate from this detailed and careful report revolve around the danger that we might become blinded 'to the larger meaning of our ideals, and may narrow

---

14   P. Kramer, *Listening to Prozac* (London: Fourth Estate, 1994).
15   B. Waters, 'Saving us from ourselves: Christology, anthropology and the seduction of posthuman medicine', in *Future Perfect?* (London: T. and T. Clark International, 2006), pp.183–95.
16   Ibid.
17   J. C. Peterson, *Genetic Turning Points: The Ethics of Human Genetic Intervention* (Grand Rapids, MI: Eerdmans, 2001).
18   Report of the President's Council on Bioethics, *Beyond Therapy*, 2003; bioethics.gov.

our sense of what it is to live, to be free, and to seek after happiness'.[19] The Council expresses deep concern that we sometimes act as though we are superhuman or divine, that we are making our bodies and minds little different from our tools, and that we risk 'flattening our souls, lowering our aspirations, and weakening our lives and attachments'.[20]

A sombre note implicit in so many of these responses is the fear that humans are attempting to improve upon God's blueprint for human life.[21] Any movement in this direction is regarded as an irreligious aspiration – aspirations that dominate theological discussions, and that may also be seen as having ill-fated ethical consequences. In my view, this type of response is based on an extreme conception of what enhancement might mean.

What is Enhancement?

The distinction usually encountered is that between enhancement and therapy. While therapy is directed towards restoring an ill person to health, enhancement generally has the connotation of improving the 'human form or functioning beyond what is necessary to sustain or restore good health'.[22] Any definition like this is far from precise. The range of possibilities is immense – from selecting embryos for specific genetic abnormalities at one extreme through to attempts at endless extension of the lifespan at the other. But what criteria are being employed for deciding the boundaries of normality and human nature and, therefore, the dimensions of therapy?

19   Ibid., p.309.
20   Ibid., p.300.
21   D. P. O'Mathuna, 'Genetic technology, enhancement, and Christian values', *The National Catholic Bioethics Quarterly* 2, 2002, pp.227–95.
22   E. T. Juengst, 'What does enhancement mean?', in *Enhancing Human Traits: Ethical and Social Implications*, ed. E. Parens (Washington DC: Georgetown University Press, 1998), pp.29–47.

Alongside these problems in defining how far therapy goes, there are problems in defining and delineating the scope of enhancement. What do we mean by enhancement? Let us consider the following analysis.[23]

Category 1 refers to the enhancement of a healthy person (H) so that they become super-healthy (SH).[24] What if we were able to protect against early onset Alzheimer's disease, coronary disease, or even mental retardation, by some form of genetic manipulation of embryos? Would such individuals in adult life be H or SH? Is this therapy or is it enhancement? They are not SH, because they are vulnerable to most diseases; they have only been protected against early onset Alzheimer's disease, heart disease or mental retardation. They have not become different forms of human being. Certainly, they may be healthier than they would otherwise have been, but they are far from illness-free or perfectly healthy. My inclination is to regard these forms of enhancement as variations of therapy, even though they are, by current standards, highly technological variants. The point here is that individuals whom we would consider today to be SH may come to be classed as normal H individuals in the future.

Changes like this are all around us. Consider the use of vaccines as prophylactics, or the widespread availability of public health measures such as the provision of clean water supplies. Uninteresting as these examples appear to us today, their 'enhancement' effects on the health of whole populations have been revolutionary. Along with dramatic increases in life expectancy and decreases in neonatal and childhood mortality, the concept of what constitutes good health has been transformed. In other words, enhancement is not simply a future phenomenon; it has already taken place in numerous societies.

Category 2 refers to enhancement that may have nothing to do with health, such as an extension of abilities. Here, enhancement encompasses those who have been endowed with super-abilities (SA), as opposed to those with the normal range of abilities (A). The SAs may be more intelligent or may have the ability to run much faster

---

23   D. G. Jones, 'Enhancement: Are ethicists excessively influenced by baseless speculations?', *Medical Humanities* 32, 2006, pp.77–81.
24   D. G. Jones, *Designers of the Future* (Oxford: Monarch, 2005).

than they would otherwise have been capable of. In these instances, rather than merely correcting defects, normal functions will have been extended.

Super-abilities may enable individuals to perform better than they would otherwise have performed – the sort of thing that worries education authorities and sports bodies. It is true that enhancements of this type may be unfair on those not in a position to benefit from them. Nevertheless, the enhanced individuals might still perform less well than other highly talented non-enhanced individuals. The bar has been raised; but is this substantially different from the way in which the bar is raised by good nutrition and hygiene, and by superior educational opportunities?

This second enhancement category is more hypothetical and futuristic than category 1. It entails pushing the 'natural' barriers more obviously than does category 1, and it has moved some distance from any health imperative.

With these thoughts in mind, we should ask where such a well-known procedure as cosmetic surgery fits in. It is not a category 1 enhancement, since it is generally unrelated to health or illness. The desire to look like someone else, to have a lighter (or darker) skin or the features of a different racial group, or to appear much younger than one's chronological age are all characteristics of category 2. Consequently, some category 2 enhancements are with us now; they do not all lie in the future.

Category 3 refers to radical transformation; the individuals are radically transformed (RT), as against those who are not transformed (NT). This is exactly what some writers have in mind when they envisage extending the lifespan to 150 years (or even 1000 years), developing hearing wavelengths previously beyond their capabilities, wiring brains directly to machines to amplify muscle movements, providing new kinds of sensory experience, or making possible various forms of telepathy. Transformations of this kind take us into the *trans-human* or *posthuman* realm.

The possibilities here seem endless, at least in the imaginations of many writers. This is because radical enhancement has no boundaries; not surprising once finitude and mortality have been overcome. Once into this realm, medicine can be used to deconstruct and reconstruct the human body. We are given to understand that posthumans will have indefinite healthy lifespans, infinite intellectual faculties, and the capability of controlling everything they are.[25] This is a world populated by visionaries and futurologists, and many legitimately ask why these thinkers are not simply ignored. The counter argument is that elements of this transformative thinking may actually be shaping the ethos of current medical practice and biomedical research.[26]

The reason for this is that regenerative medicine is repeatedly looked to as a means of greatly extending longevity, with humans living much longer and also maintaining their physical and mental capabilities throughout their whole lifespan. This is based on the presumption that ageing is a disease, and can therefore be treated and even vanquished. The goal of medicine is transformed into a means of waging war against death. Mortality will be replaced by immortality, endlessly renewed bodies in an age- and disease-free world. Extreme and uninformed as these ideas might appear, this is a realm of discourse that has infiltrated social, theological and even ethical debate. What, after all of this, are we to make of therapy and enhancement?

This is where the problem lies. Having rejected these extreme scenarios, some move immediately to a rejection of any interventions in the genome or brain. This is the stance of the bioconservatives.[27] They call for this total rejection because any use of technology to improve the quality of life or of mental functioning can be viewed as part of a much broader endeavour – that of extending the lifespan indefinitely or giving individuals unlimited mental powers. No room has now been left for category 1 measures, which are viewed solely in terms of the far more radical and idealistic goals of category 3. The underlying assumption is that the ethos of medical practice and research has already been transformed: instead of caring for patients, its only interest is in curing people of every conceivable malady, up to and including ageing and death.

Once medicine is seen in these terms, the implications for ethics are enormous. This is because human embryo research, using PGD or

25   N. Bostrom, 'In defense of posthuman dignity', *Bioethics* 19, 2005, pp.202–14.
26   Waters, 'Saving us from ourselves'.
27   Bostrom, 'In defense of posthuman dignity'.

embryonic stem cells, regenerative medicine, and the use of psycho-pharmaceuticals in psychiatric conditions have all become part of a posthuman agenda. Not surprisingly, they are assessed negatively by those who find this agenda a troublesome one.[28] They are viewed as little more than forms of illicit enhancement. No room is left for looking into these procedures in their own right; they have become submerged beneath a welter of fanciful aspirations, most of which are so far removed from scientific reality as to constitute impenetrable hurdles to serious ethical (or theological) debate.

Let us stop to consider the two major challenges raised by these considerations. How do we know when we have passed from therapy into enhancement, let alone from one category of enhancement into another? How can we distinguish between the ethical dimensions of a procedure as routine as PGD and a visionary procedure such as designing a tailor-made baby?

Making Important Distinctions

So often it is assumed that the distinction between therapy and enhancement is clearly defined; similarly with the distinctions between normality and abnormality, and health and disease. The assumption also appears to be made that, whatever these distinctions might be, they are unchanging. They are the same today as they were in 1950 or 1850, or they are the same now across all societies.

Routinely accepted biological limits are wide, and the concept of normality is broad and tenuous. Psychopharmaceuticals can be used to combat everything from shyness and forgetfulness to sleepiness and depression. Are any of these diseases? Is depression normal? Clinical depression may be a disease entity, but what about the low-grade, sub-clinical depression that afflicts so many people? If it is not a clinical phenomenon, and therefore not an illness, is treatment with drugs a form of enhancement? No matter how we respond to these questions,

28   Jones, 'Enhancement'.

we have to ask whether there is any virtue in living with low-grade depression if it can be ameliorated? What is normal? In a similar vein, should we treat hyperactivity in children who are difficult to handle? Are their behaviours normal or abnormal? Does Ritalin administration have a role as part of a genuine therapeutic regime or is it a form of social manipulation? The line between the normal and the pathological can be a very fine one indeed. And we may be far from sure which side of the line we are on.

And what about the slight deterioration in memory that ordinarily accompanies ageing, demonstrated by minor forgetfulness in everyday activities? This is sometimes referred to as age-associated memory impairment. Is this normal or abnormal? Should it be viewed as no more than an interesting phenomenon, or is it a mild disease state? Alternatively, it may be nothing more than a syndrome dreamed up by the pharmaceutical industry. This is not simply a matter of abstract theorising, since mild memory losses may be a prelude to mild cognitive impairment and ultimately to the dementia of Alzheimer's disease. But, of course, they might not. There is no questioning the pathology of the latter, nor the therapeutic rationale for its treatment. At the present time, the early stages are almost inevitably shrouded in a therapy/enhancement fog.[29]

In the other direction, drugs influencing memory could prove useful in younger age-groups, where boosting test scores at school and university would be the driving force. This brings us face-to-face with the concerns of the affluent 'worried well', aided and abetted by commercial pressures within the pharmaceutical industry.[30] Such a use of memory-enhancing drugs appears close to a category 1 enhancement measure. It also highlights how society's values and desires can shape the direction and interpretation of scientific endeavour.

It is impossible to escape the blurred nature of the normal/ abnormal, and therapy/enhancement boundaries, a blurring that becomes even more problematic when a time element is introduced. Expectations of what constitutes good health and normal life expec-

---

29   Ibid.
30   C. Arnst, 'I can't remember', *Business Week*, 1 September 2003; http://www. businessweek.com.

tancy have changed out of all recognition since the early years of the twentieth century. Moreover, our expectations bear no resemblance to those of many people today living in the two-thirds world. Are our expectations normal, or are theirs? If some form of direct intervention on the functioning of the brains of those with early stage Alzheimer's disease were to be developed over the next ten years, would that be therapy or enhancement? If it were to be classed as therapy, it would represent a return to good health unimaginable today, let alone in 1990 or 1950. Or, if it were seen as enhancement, would it be an enhancement to be welcomed, or one to be feared and rejected? I would suggest it would be a category 1 enhancement with enormous potential for good. What this tells us is that the dimensions of normality, health and therapy are never static, and their borders will always be blurred. Definitions are inevitably time and place dependent.

It is a pity that discussions of posthumanism are generally seen as concerning the future, the assumption appearing to be that we ourselves are unenhanced. However, this is fallacious. Technological interventions into the human condition did not commence in the latter years of the twentieth century. Compared with the hunter-gatherers we must seem like posthumans;[31] or, if this is an overstatement, that we have at least been dramatically enhanced. The ethical challenges facing us would have been totally foreign to earlier generations, let alone the hunter-gatherers, but this is not sufficient reason to regret the technological developments wrought by our predecessors.

The indefinite borderlands between therapy and enhancement, and even within enhancement, lead to the conclusion that these designations provide far from definitive ethical guideposts. Both of the terms 'therapy' and 'enhancement' are far too imprecise to be helpful by themselves. Resnik came to a similar conclusion when he wrote:

> Genetic enhancement is not inherently immoral nor is genetic therapy inherently moral. Some forms of enhancement are immoral, others are not; likewise, some types of therapy are immoral, others are not.[32]

31   Bostrom, 'In defense of posthuman dignity'.
32   D. B. Resnik, 'The moral significance of the therapy-enhancement distinction in human genetics', *Cambridge Quarterly of Healthcare Ethics* 9, 2000, pp. 365–77.

Each case has to be examined on its own merits. A simple label of 'therapy' or 'enhancement' will never provide the answer.

Ongoing Concerns

But there may still be problems. Many think that there are, since in their eyes the medical enterprise is being irremediably damaged by incipient enhancement techniques of the radically transformative type. We are being dragged into category 3, whether we like it or not.

Pellegrino defines enhancement as an intervention that goes beyond the ends of medicine as traditionally conceived,[33] and he sees this as part of the medicalisation of every facet of human existence. He regrets the manner in which physicians are becoming enhancement therapists, devoted to increasing the alleged happiness of patients rather than seeking to heal them. In his view, enhancement provides hopes for an earthly paradise for those who no longer believe in an after-life. The inner core of medicine has been transformed by what Pellegrino regards as illicit enhancement which is precipitating a cataclysmic reinterpretation of medical therapy.[34]

Alongside these concerns, Pellegrino concludes that enhancement aimed at ends such as the desire for healthy, bright and lovable children is understandable.[35] It may also be acceptable on condition that the means to bring these states about do not dehumanise their subjects. Over against this, enhancement focusing on the thrills of going farther and faster in athletics becomes an end in itself. It is this latter form that he views as beyond the healing ends of medicine. These two contrasting modes of enhancement are illustrations of categories 1 and 2 respectively.

33   E. D. Pellegrino, 'Biotechnology, human enhancement, and the ends of medicine', *Dignity* 10, 2004, pp.1–5.
34   Ibid.
35   Ibid.

Related concerns at the beginning of human life centre on the drive towards perfection. Sandel, for one, views with apprehension what he regards as the drift towards mastery, with its associated ethic of wilfulness, leading to 'hyperparenting'.[36] He is alarmed by what he interprets as the hubris of designing parents, seeking to master the mystery of birth. Sandel wishes us to retain an ethic of giftedness, appreciating children as gifts, and rejecting enhancement aimed at perfection.[37] This leads to a rejection of wilfulness and dominion, in favour of giftedness, reverence and beholding. He writes:

> There is something appealing, even intoxicating, about a vision of human freedom unfettered by the given. ... It is often assumed that the powers of enhancement we now possess arose as an inadvertent by-product of biomedical progress ... to cure disease. ... It is more plausible to view genetic engineering as the ultimate expression of our resolve to see ourselves astride the world, the masters of our nature ... but ... it threatens to banish our appreciation of life as a gift ...

As with a number of other writers, Sandel is unwilling to separate the grand vistas from conventional medical practice. For me, on the other hand, these vistas do not appear as inevitable concomitants of the entry of technology into the reproductive process. Nevertheless, his stress on the ethic of giftedness, and on openness to the unbidden, with his critique of excessive mastery, dominion and wilfulness, are salutary lessons that we would be unwise to ignore. While they do not provide clear directions through the enhancement maze, their negative facets do have a bearing on enhancements in categories 1 or 2, and not just on those in category 3.[38]

The central concern of writers such as Pellegrino and Sandel is the prospect of descending into eugenics. But is the notion of eugenics unhelpful in its unrealistic thrust? Desirable traits such as intelligence, height and appearance are polygenic and are exceptionally difficult to manipulate. Even if a number of genes were isolated that influenced,

36   M. J. Sandel, 'The case against perfection', *The Atlantic Monthly* 293, 2004, pp.51–62.

37   Ibid.

38   Jones, 'Enhancement'.

say, intelligence, the eventual transformation would probably only be in the order of a few IQ points. The manipulation of an embryo by the addition of 'smart' genes or 'beautiful' genes would be incomprehensibly difficult.

Even if such scientific hurdles were to be overcome, we would inevitably be disappointed with the results of genetic enhancement, for genes are no more than one facet of the myriad processes that make up a person. The environment, whether prenatal, social, nutritional, educational or parental, has an equally large influence on the final 'product' as have the genes.

I have sympathy with those whose concerns stem from posthuman excesses. However, enormous care is required to ensure that these philosophical dimensions are not used as weapons against clinical and scientific aspirations that fit far more readily within a conventional therapeutic context or, at the most, a category 1 enhancement context.

What does Theology Bring to the Enhancement Debate?

Theologians are right to be concerned about some aspects of the enhancement debate. There are extremes around, and they should be combated. John Harris, Professor of Bioethics at the University of Manchester, has recently argued that we have a moral imperative to extend both the human lifespan and the quality of human life. We should develop technologies to extend human life for as long as conceivably possible.[39] While claims like this can be interpreted in a variety of ways, with different outcomes, one can appreciate why theologians might be concerned. Arguments of this nature tend to view human life in solely material terms: human life is nothing more than bodily life and material existence; hence, length of life becomes

---

39   M. Henderson, 'Scientists have "moral duty" to help us live beyond 100', *The Times*, 13 March 2006; www.timesonline.co.uk.

the centrepiece of human aspirations. What, then, might constitute a theological approach?

An interesting starting point is provided by Hanson, when he writes that a Christian perspective:

> ... affirms the inherent goodness of creation, and diagnoses the 'defects' in the human situation in terms of sin. The result is a very different way of thinking about the prospect of human enhancement and what it might mean. It suggests that enhancement technologies and the values that motivate then must be approached with suspicion.[40]

Hanson's suspicion prompts him to delineate a number of religious benchmarks by which enhancement technologies might be judged. He wishes to resist the idea that to be finite is to suffer, since this would mean that the contingency of creation is held in contempt. Allied with this is his opposition to technologies that express a 'will-to-power' over conditions of finiteness, rather than being a faithful response to suffering. A further evaluation follows from this: asking whether the technologies in question interfere with humanity's dual nature of free-dom and finiteness, and therefore with the ability to recognise both the goodness and the evils of humanity. Finally, he concludes that tech-nologies that promote complicity with norms of narcissism, vanity and self-sufficiency, that is, with sinful pride, are problematic.

General as these considerations are, they serve as useful pointers for any theological perspective. In themselves they do not preclude any particular modifications, which are to be assessed using the cat-egories I have outlined. Nevertheless, they serve to direct us away from the catastrophic posthuman framework of so many theological contributions, towards one that takes seriously what is actually happening in scientific laboratories.

Deane-Drummond is correct when she expresses her scepticism about the use of salvific language on the part of scientists, since it promises far too much.[41] Nevertheless, it also behoves theologians to move beyond negative responses to this extremism. For her, it is far

---

40   M. J. Hanson, 'Indulging anxiety: Human enhancement from a Protestant perspective', *Christian Bioethics* 5, 1999, pp.121–38, p.127.
41   Deane-Drummond, 'How might a virtue ethic ...?'

more valuable to explore theological strands based on wisdom and prudence, with important motifs being provided by humility and weakness. It is right to be cautious, but this by itself does not lead to outright opposition to all forms of exploratory therapy and the modest categories of enhancement.[42] In our concern to respond to the overweening ambitions of some scientists and thinkers, we should not succumb to the temptation to bless the status quo as if it were perfect. The status quo is far from that; indeed, it is frequently filled with human misery, some of which is genetically caused.[43]

It would be a shame if Christians finished up inadvertently defending the status quo and the present state of biomedical understanding and control for fear of some highly speculative posthumanist scenarios. There are ways of working towards a better future that are far more modest than that predicated on a posthumanist agenda, and that take serious account of theologically helpful pointers. Those working within a framework of faith should be prepared to embrace joyfully category 1 and at least some category 2 enhancements, while vigorously arguing against category 3 varieties with their veneer of posthumanism.

We need to ensure that we develop a paradigm that leaves room for the serious discussion of ethical issues around stem cell research and therapy, PGD, and gene therapy, where the focus is on possible clinical applications (either now or in the future). Whether one labels some of these as enhancements or therapy is of little relevance to medical treatment, where patients capable of benefiting from the procedures are the objects of attention.

But am I ignoring the power of present day science, or failing to consider sufficiently seriously the future directions of science? Maybe I am. However, the line between where science is today and where it will be in 30 years' time (let alone 300 years' time) will probably be a tortuous one. Future-scoping exercises are fraught with uncertainties and have a poor track record. As little as 30 to 40 years ago, discussions of reproductive cloning concentrated on the manner in which

---

42   Peterson, *Genetic Turning Points.*
43   T. Peters, *Playing God? Genetic Determinism and Human Freedom* (New York: Routledge, 2003).

it would result in the redirection of human evolution; no thought was given to its role in agriculture and the pharmaceutical industry.

The scientific enterprise, of its very essence, is a creative one, aiming to find new ways of addressing medical and allied problems. Its approach to problems is, however, of a strictly limited nature, driven as it is by its reductionist methodology. In no senses is this antagonistic to the giftedness of life, even when the realm is the reproductive one. Indeed, as has been pointed out by Parens, in discussing the gratitude and creativity frameworks the two emphases should be held in tension:

> As one side emphasizes our obligation to remember that life is a gift and that we need to learn to let things be, the other emphasizes our obligation to transform that gift and to exhibit our creativity.[44]

The challenge is to hold these two in tension, something which many feel is not currently being achieved, particularly in those areas where the science is driven by pharmaceutical and commercial interests. I accept this, but do not accept that this is an argument against the creative impulse within science. Viewing scientific investigations as part of a posthuman agenda will not solve any challenges that lie at the border between therapy and enhancement, whether one seeks to prohibit or advocate them.

Discussion of enhancement would be more helpful if we could accept that we *are* enhanced, at least at the category 1 level. Ethical discussion could then be grounded in the present, and not in some unclear and largely untenable future. We could then see that fundamental moral values, such as the benefit of the individual, justice and fairness, are central, no matter what is contemplated – be it therapy or enhancement.

While theological considerations do not provide specific answers about what is or is not acceptable, they do serve to provide a framework by which it is possible to accept our finiteness and mortality. While acceptance of realities like these could lead to fatalism, also

---

44   E. Parens, 'Authenticity and ambivalence: Towards understanding the enhancement debate', *Hastings Center Report* 35, 2005, pp.34–41.

integral to the Christian faith is awareness of the magnificence and grandeur of human beings. It is the duality of these characteristics that leads to scientific achievements as we know them, together with a humility regarding their vast but limited dimensions. In these terms, enhancement technologies can be assessed and critiqued, valuing and utilising those that appear to advance human welfare, whilst arguing against those whose aspirations appear to be counterproductive.

D. GARETH JONES

Is PGD a Form of Eugenics?

Introduction

It is difficult to overestimate the seismic effects that *in vitro* fertilisation (IVF) has had on the societies in which we live. Its use in bypassing infertility has been overshadowed by the many other uses to which it can be put in transforming the reproductive process for those wishing to have children with same-sex partners, timing precisely when children will be born, or even delaying this until after menopause. These and other consequences of IVF depend upon one overriding ability, namely, the ability to investigate and manipulate human embryos in the laboratory. The human embryo has ceased to be a mysterious and unfathomable entity, and this is the root of the disquiet expressed by many when confronted by techniques for controlling embryonic development.

Control of our earliest beginnings is equated with control of our lives as human beings; all our fears stemming from the latter form of control are expressed in the form of opposition to the former type of control. And so it is that pre-implantation genetic diagnosis (PGD), an offshoot of IVF, encapsulates the fears of many over eugenics. In the eyes of many, the horrors of eugenics that came to a head in the 1930s and 1940s in Nazi Germany have re-emerged with PGD.

PGD is a procedure devised to test early human embryos for serious inherited genetic conditions. Only embryos that are free from the condition are transferred to a woman, in the expectation that a normal pregnancy will result. Inevitably, this involves selecting embryos: selecting those that are not genetic carriers of the disease trait, and discarding those that have the gene responsible for the disease. Herein lies the perceived problem: *selection*. Some embryos are chosen for further development; others are not. Some will be given the chance of becoming a new human being; others will be denied that chance. Some will become like you and me; others will be discarded. Perhaps one can envision two classes of embryos, the privileged and the underprivileged. It is easy for us to get carried away with such descriptions, and yet the reality is far more prosaic.

The Science of PGD

PGD can only be used in conjunction with IVF, even when there is no evidence of infertility. During PGD, those embryos found to have a serious genetic condition are discarded. This is the current extent to which selection is involved. When PGD is undertaken, the live birth rate per embryo transfer is around 20 per cent,[1] not dissimilar to the live birth rate for IVF in the United Kingdom.[2]

The first live births of healthy babies after PGD analysis occurred in the early 1990s. Since then PGD has been used increasingly in the detection of three types of abnormalities: single gene disorders, familial sex-linked disorders and familial chromosomal disorders. In addition, it is being used increasingly for nonfamilial chromosomal disorders associated with advanced reproductive age, where there may be specific numerical chromosomal disorders, including Down syndrome. Some examples of disorders for which PGD may be used are:

Single gene disorders:
- Cystic fibrosis
- Huntington's disease

1   J. C. Harper, K. Boelaert and J. Geraedts, ESHRE PGD Consortium data collection V: 'Cycles from January to December 2002 with pregnancy follow-up to October 2003', *Human Reproduction* 21, 2006, pp.3−21.

2   HFEA, 'New HFEA Guide to infertility shows birth rates following IVF treatment continue to increase', press release in conjunction with the release of the 2006−07 HFEA Guide to Infertility. Available from the Human Fertilisation and Embryology Authority: http://www.hfea.gov.uk/PressOffice/Archive/1149 194953. Accessed 7 June 2006.

- Myotonic dystrophy
- Sickle cell anaemia
- Spinal muscular atrophy
- Thalassaemia

Sex-linked disorders:
- Duchenne's muscular dystrophy
- Haemophilia
- Fragile-X syndrome

Chromosomal disorders:
- Patau syndrome (trisomy 13 syndrome)
- Prader–Willi syndrome

A further use for PGD is where there is repeated reproductive failure, such as recurrent implantation failure and miscarriage.

PGD involves the extraction of one or two cells (blastomeres) from the very early embryo, when it is between four to eight cells; this can also be done at the blastocyst stage, when the embryo is five days old. The extracted cells are then tested, via one of two methods, for the presence of chromosomal or gene disorders.

PGD was first developed using polymerase chain reaction (PCR). Today PCR is generally used to detect single gene defects, although, when PGD was first developed, it was used to detect the Y chromosome for sex-linked disorders. PCR allows for the creation of many copies of pieces of DNA coding for the gene under investigation. These can then be examined for the presence of genetic mutations. The misdiagnosis rate for PCR is very low.[3]

Fluorescent *in situ* hybridisation (FISH) is a process in which the extracted blastomeres are incubated with chromosomal-specific DNA probes, which have a fluorescent marker attached. By using fluorescence microscopy, coloured spots can be detected on the sample, which enables the easy identification of chromosomal abnormalities. For example, a normal probe of chromosome 21 results in a sample with two spots; in contrast, three spots are visible in Down syndrome.

3   Harper et al., ESHRE PGD Consortium data collection V.

Testing for numerical errors in chromosomes like this is an illustration
of aneuploidy screening. FISH is employed to determine the sex of
embryos where sex-linked conditions are suspected, and also to detect
structural chromosomal abnormalities and aneuploidies. The rate of
misdiagnosis for FISH is also very low.[4]

PGD was initially offered only to couples with genetic predispositions to certain conditions. Currently, however, there are many
PGD clinics also offering aneuploidy screening to couples who are
having trouble conceiving or carrying a baby. This is because this type
of screening appears to improve the live birth rate for couples with
fertility problems.[5]

At present it is not possible to screen for all 46 chromosomes
using PGD. Between nine and eleven chromosomes can be tested at
the moment. Therefore, even if an embryo is replaced on the assumption that there are no numerical abnormalities on the chromosomes
tested, there is still a possibility that one or more of the remaining
chromosomes are affected. However, with the present rate of scientific
developments, it might not be long before the ability to test all 46
chromosomes is achieved.

Extending PGD

One of the features of PGD is that it enables the sex of embryos to be
readily determined. This is both an advantage and a disadvantage. The
advantage is that, when dealing with sex-linked genetic conditions, it
enables embryos of the appropriate sex to be selected so that the
resulting child will not suffer from the condition in question. The
disadvantage is that sex selection can be used for social control of the
next generation by providing parents with a child of the preferred sex.

---

4   Ibid.
5   S. Munné, J. Fischer, A. Warner et al., 'Preimplantation genetic diagnosis sig-
     nificantly reduces pregnancy loss in infertile couples: a multicenter study',
     Fertility and Sterility 85, 2006, pp.326–32.

This form of sex selection has nothing to do with anything medical or therapeutic, but it does illustrate the paper-thin boundary between medical and social drivers.

A further use to which PGD may be put is the avoidance of the implantation of an embryo with a late onset genetic disorder, such as Huntington's disease, or one with a predisposition to develop conditions such as diabetes, high blood pressure, breast cancer, or even – hypothetically – Alzheimer's disease.

In the UK, the Human Fertilisation and Embryology Authority (HFEA) has recently allowed the use of PGD for lower penetrance, later onset inherited conditions, such as breast, bowel and ovarian cancer.[6] This has been extremely contentious, since the new individual would not suffer from any disease for many years. Not only this, the individual might never have actually developed the condition in question. This is because one is dealing here with lower penetrance conditions. In other words, embryos are being selected against because of the *possibility* that future individuals might suffer from a particular condition. Can this truly be described as therapy, or is it taking therapy into unforeseen realms that have little in common with any conventional medical practice? It appears to involve the destruction of embryos *just in case* a future individual will suffer from a particular disease.

Another term to have entered our vocabularies over recent times is 'saviour sibling'. In this, one baby is brought into the world in an attempt to save the life of an already existing sibling (with, say, Franconi's anaemia). For many people, this produces even more moral antibodies, since it appears to be using one child for the benefit of another. Some argue that this is exploitation of the worst kind.

Technically, it is human leukocyte antigen (HLA) tissue typing, which is an additional step to PGD to determine if an embryo could lead to the birth of a child who is a tissue match for an ill sibling. PGD is used to select embryos that are free of the familial disorder in question and are also a tissue match for the older sibling. This double

6   HFEA, 'HFEA Authority decision'; available from: http://www.hfea.gov.uk/ AboutHFEA/HFEAPolicy/Choicesandboundaries/TheAuthoritydecision/t0JCK FY6.pdf. Accessed 18 May 2006.

requirement of embryos means that more embryos are discarded than in straightforward PGD, including embryos known to be biologically normal (those free of the disorder but not a tissue match). At birth, the umbilical cord blood of this newborn child will probably be used to treat the ill older sibling.

Here, the concerns revolve around the way in which the resulting child is regarded. If the child were to be perceived as little more than an 'organ farm' for the ill sibling, no justification could possibly be found for moving in this direction. On the other hand, if the child is treated with as much care and love as the ill sibling, and if they are given every opportunity to develop and be themselves, it is far more difficult to see what basic ethical values have been abrogated. Of course, for those who oppose the selection of embryos as a matter of principle, there will be no place for going down the 'saviour sibling' path; the double selection will be more objectionable than the single selection of PGD by itself.

Beginning to Unravel PGD

Before looking specifically at the relationship between PGD and eugenics, it is important to consider some of the general features of PGD, since these lay the groundwork for the assessment of any eugenic implications.

In the first place, PGD is not a panacea for all the ills of either humanity or individuals, even our genetic ills. It is necessary to reiterate such an obvious statement, since the ethical literature is awash with vast generalisations concerning either the redemptive or abusive powers of any form of genetic selection. PGD should be seen for what it is: another means of partially tackling certain genetic conditions, limited in scope, even if associated with considerable potential. It will always be ethically ambiguous, and this has to be recognised by society, equally by those who welcome what it might bring and by those who fear its possibilities.

From this follows a second issue. We must never be tempted to look to PGD to provide us with perfectly healthy children. Idealistic expectations like this are deceptive, since they suggest there is a norm to which all children must conform. Unfortunately, this medical aspiration is a very easy ideal to which to succumb, since contained within it is the desire to do the best for our children. Such a worthy goal is difficult to refute, until it is realised that it is an unmanageable one on the purely medical front, as well as involving rejection of what we are as human beings. Accepting and loving our children, wanting the best for them and hoping to see them flourish in all aspects of their lives; these aspirations have nothing to do with seeking genetic perfection.

A third issue that should not be overlooked is the doubly artificial nature of PGD. As we have seen, it can only be carried out following IVF. Hence, when contemplating PGD, what one is faced with is IVF-plus-PGD. This has two consequences. Reproduction has become a seriously laboratory-based exercise, which will not, in all likelihood, be undertaken for anything other than pressing reasons. Associated with this is its cost, since both IVF and PGD are expensive technical undertakings. Most people will not be able to afford this, especially if the grounds for moving in this direction are insubstantial. Even for good reasons, there would need to be extensive government support, and this raises a plethora of funding issues for all health service providers.

Will future generations look back positively on PGD, or will it be seen as a slippery slope to sex selection for superficial reasons, to unwarranted manipulation of human embryos, and in a eugenic direction? We do not know, and science alone will not provide an answer. Ongoing ethical reflection, informed by precise science, is needed to balance the prospects for good against what seem to be the dangers.

Selection: The Central Paradigm of PGD

Inevitably, PGD involves selecting embryos: selecting those that are not genetic carriers of the disease trait, and discarding those that have the gene responsible for the disease. Certain embryos are chosen; other embryos are rejected. Put like this, it is not difficult to appreciate why PGD so readily acquires theological overtones: chosen and rejected, in the way in which God is sometimes depicted as choosing and rejecting. Against this backdrop, how can we possibly allow mere humans to choose some and reject others? The theological thrust becomes even more pressing when embryos are equated with people; it is not embryos that are chosen and rejected, but people like us, who are either set on the way to life or consigned to early destruction. While only some will argue in this manner, this gives a feel for the emotional drives behind their rejection of PGD.

Consequently, PGD is anathema to some people. For those to whom all embryos are human persons (in the sense in which those of us reading these words are human persons, and all embryos are to be treated as of equal value), one embryo should never be selected over and above another embryo in this manner. And yet it is well known that, while some embryos are routinely selected under natural conditions, others are discarded. Although such selection is not under human control, it is occurring all the time. It is more than likely that everyone who is born started life as an embryo that emerged as a result of a natural process of selection, in the sense that a number of embryos with chromosomal or genetic abnormalities would have been discarded prior to the successful implantation of this one embryo.

It is generally accepted that there is a vast natural wastage of very early embryos: up to 70 per cent.[7] Current information from IVF suggests that, of those embryos that appear to be usable on day 3 (that is, those where there is a fast cleavage rate of cells and few cell fragments), only around 50 to 70 per cent are still usable at the

---

7   N. S. Macklon, J. P. Geraedis and B. C. Fauser, 'Conception to ongoing pregnancy: the "black box" of early pregnancy loss', *Human Reproduction Update* 8, 2002, pp.333–43.

blastocyst stage about three days later. Most embryos stop developing because they have chromosomal abnormalities. While it is notoriously difficult to obtain reliable estimates of the figures, probably 70 per cent or so of all embryos have such abnormalities. For women in their 40s, the figure probably rises to over 90 per cent. This is part of the human condition, and is a major reason why fertile women have only a 20 to 30 per cent chance of becoming pregnant in any one month.

This is a form of embryo selection in which the embryos chosen are those that appear to be 'fit' to proceed throughout gestation. Some are fit to survive; others are not. While what happens naturally cannot, by itself, be used as an argument about what is ethically permissible in the laboratory, neither can it be completely ignored. PGD, as I have described it, is doing essentially the same thing. True, the laboratory intervention is extending the choices that are being made, but these choices are in basically the same direction as that which occurs naturally. There is no reason that this should always be the case (and the 'saviour sibling' scenario is a case in point), but it is true of the thrust of most PGD as we currently know it.

Before moving beyond fertility clinics, it is useful to remind ourselves that embryos are routinely selected in IVF. This has nothing to do with PGD. The normality of embryos is used to determine which embryos to implant in a woman's uterus during IVF treatment and which to discard. This is usually the distinction that is made between viable and non-viable embryos, those that appear to have the characteristics to enable them to continue to develop normally, and those that lack these characteristics. There is no hint in these decisions that some embryos are preferable to others on the basis of what they will ultimately become. The choice is entirely whether they have prospects of developing any further. Nevertheless, selection is taking place.

Outside the reproductive area, we routinely select one person over another – in education, health, or employment. Selection takes place when we pick one school rather than another for our children; selection occurs in adoption when a child with one set of characteristics is preferred over one with another set; selection is evident when we choose one person to be our partner rather than another. These and many other illustrations of selection affect the lives of other human beings (sometimes detrimentally), and yet we regard them as ethically and theologically valid. Selecting student A over student B for a highly sought-after university course will have implications for both students, and perhaps negative ones for student B. Similarly, selecting patient C over patient D to have an expensive and much needed operation may result in extending the life (or quality of life) of person C but not that of D. Nevertheless, we consider this acceptable as long as the criteria underlying the selection are valid and equitable. Hence, selection *per se* should not be used as an argument or weapon against the selection of one embryo over another.

But is selection at the beginning of human life different in character from all such illustrations of postnatal selection? Are these latter less determinative and perhaps less devastating, and do they interfere less with the essence of the person? The crux of the difference is that selection at the embryonic stage is that of existence versus non-existence, whereas postnatal selection simply modifies an existing person. Both are examples of human control. The thrust of embryonic selection is positive, in that it is to produce an individual who will be free of a debilitating condition. It is not to end the life of an individual. Nevertheless, all forms of selection (both embryonic and postnatal) have pitfalls. In the case of PGD, we have to ask how selection is being used. Many of the diseases currently tested for are devastating in their effects, and the pain and suffering of those with the conditions (and of their families) is enormous. However, some of the conditions that are tested for are not necessarily in this category. For example, some syndromes can result in relatively minor impairment. For other conditions the onset of the disease does not take place until later in life, for example Huntington's disease, which usually occurs when the individual is between 30 and 45 years of age. Hence, the selection against Huntington's disease is a decision that a mid-life illness, debilitating when it sets in, is reason enough to select against embryos.

This demonstrates that selection in PGD is far from ethically neutral, but neither is any other form of selection. Individuals and societies make wrong choices. Selection can be on ephemeral grounds, and this is widespread. Consequently, it would not be surprising if this were also to occur with PGD. But, as I have indicated, the rigours and costs associated with PGD may limit the more extravagant uses of it.

Nevertheless, selection remains, and this leads to the claim that PGD has a eugenics rationale. Is PGD inherently eugenicist in its orientation? If not, how far is it from such a perspective?

Eugenics: What is It?

The mere mention of eugenics calls forth recollections of the atrocities performed in Nazi Germany. But eugenics was not just a product of the Nazi regime; such movements were widespread in many countries during the first half of the twentieth century. Those eugenics movements saw the practice of both positive and negative eugenics. Positive eugenics was highlighted by the 'fitter families' campaign in the USA, which sought to bring about the increased production of genetically desirable children by those with 'good genes'. Over and against this, negative eugenics involved the forced sterilisation of those with undesirable genetic characteristics; in some places this was interpreted broadly, so as to include those with mental, physical and psychological disabilities, habitual criminals and 'moral perverts'.[8]

Definitions of eugenics abound, the variety of which is self-defeating. Francis Galton, who coined the term, defined it as 'the science of improving inherited stock, not only by judicious matings, but by all the influences which give the more suitable strains a better chance'.[9] Thus the traditional understanding of eugenics was that, by selective breeding, those with 'good' genes could produce more children and thus improve the gene pool, while those with 'bad' genes had few children, or none at all. Along these lines, the Oxford English Dictionary has at times past defined eugenics as 'the production of fine (esp. human) offspring by improvement of inherited qualities'.[10]

8   D. Galton, *In Our Own Image* (London: Little, Brown and Company, 2001).
9   Francis Galton, quoted in D. J. Galton and C. J. Galton, 'Francis Galton and eugenics today', *Journal of Medical Ethics* 24, 1998, pp.99–105.
10   *The Concise Oxford Dictionary of Current English*, 6th edn, ed. J. B. Sykes (Oxford: OUP, 1976).

Modern definitions are more eclectic. Some define eugenics in terms of a particular movement at the beginning of the twentieth century. Others are extremely broad; witness the following, with its view that any reproductive choice is eugenic in nature:

> Parental eugenics occurs every time people select mates or sperm or egg donors. ... Most parents do not make their reproductive choices with the sole aim of controlling the human gene pool; any effects these choices have on the gene pool are unintended consequences of parental actions.[11]

One writer discussing the change in the understanding of eugenics has observed that, 'while eugenics was originally defined in terms of an outcome – the improvement of society's gene pool – its contemporary usage is generally in terms of a process.'[12] The same writer defines the contemporary understanding of eugenics as being:

> the notion of human beings exerting control over which genes are transmitted from one generation to the next – irrespective of whether it is society or the prospective parents exerting the control, and irrespective of whether the action will have any effect on the gene pool.[13]

The theologian Deane-Drummond, discussing eugenics in relation to modern medical practice, writes:

> I suggest that what has persisted in both the eugenics of the last century and more recent contemporary medical practice, including reformulated versions of eugenics ... is the view that there are those in the population whom society would be better off without. Hence, while in most cases genetic screening would not be 'eugenic' in the sense of being an effective means of removing genes from a population, it is eugenic in as much as it assumes that there are undesirables in our midst.[14]

11   D. B. Resnik, 'The moral significance of the therapy–enhancement distinction in human genetics', *Cambridge Quarterly of Healthcare Ethics* 9, 2000, pp. 365–77.
12   D. W. Jordaan, 'Preimplantation genetic screening and selection: An ethical analysis', *Biotechnology Law Report* 6, 2003, pp.586–601.
13   Ibid.
14   C. Deane-Drummond, *Genetics and Christian Ethics* (Cambridge: CUP, 2006).

It may be that eugenics itself can be subdivided into acceptable and unacceptable eugenics. Consider the following:

> We suggest it is more accurate to see modern clinical genetics as a natural development of an existing eugenic thrust in society, rather than as something that now threatens to produce a new eugenic society.[15]

Perhaps a eugenic thrust is endemic to much that medicine aspires to, but this has nothing in common with the goals of the eugenics movement of a hundred or so years ago, and certainly not with the horrors of the Nazi era. Attractive as this distinction is, there is no agreement on it. For some, any manipulation of the gene pool is regarded as automatically evil. For others it is possible to have 'good' eugenics, which has little in common with the actions undertaken during the earlier part of the twentieth century.

This diversity of viewpoints on what constitutes eugenics raises serious questions about the value of attempting to decide whether or not PGD (or any other procedure for that matter) is eugenic in its thrust. It all depends on one's definition of eugenics.

Regardless of these disagreements, it is generally accepted that it is the element of *coercion* that makes eugenics particularly distasteful. It was the enforced sterilisation of 'undesirables' in the first half of the twentieth century that condemns that form of eugenics. Were PGD, or any other form of reproductive decision making, to be mandated by the state, thereby removing freedom of choice and autonomy, it would rapidly assume all the negative overtones of coercive eugenics. But what if this is not the case?

15 M. H. Parker, L. F. Kevin and R. Findlay, 'Eugenics or empowered choice? Community issues arising from prenatal testing', *The Australian and New Zealand Journal of Obstetrics and Gynecology* 42, 2002, pp.10–14.

Eugenicist Overtones to PGD?

In order to explore this question let us look at a number of scenarios.

Scenario 1

During routine IVF the embryologist has to decide whether embryos are viable or non-viable. She decides on routine grounds, and transfers one embryo to the uterus, freezes three more embryos for possible use in future, and discards two embryos that show no signs of developing normally. She considered four to be viable at this early stage, and two to be non-viable. A selection has been made. Any eugenic overtones are minimal, but there has been selection.

Scenario 2

PGD is undertaken because the parents wish to avoid having another child with cystic fibrosis. Two embryos are found to have the gene responsible for cystic fibrosis, and are discarded. The third embryo studied does not have this gene, it is viable, and is transferred to the uterus. There are eugenicist overtones, since if there were not, the first embryos found to be viable would have been transferred even if they had carried the gene for cystic fibrosis. Are these overtones acceptable? Should PGD used in this way be called eugenics, and compared with classical eugenics? There is no coercion, since the parents did not have to use PGD. The intention is a therapeutic one, in that their aim is to have a healthy child. However, in order to achieve this, some embryos will have been selected against. Is this an extension of what happens naturally, or is it an illustration of maleficent human intervention?

Scenario 3

PGD is again undertaken, this time in the knowledge that a particular genetically-determined type of breast cancer might be present in any female embryos. There is a compelling clinical history of breast cancer in this family, in that four of the mother's close relatives have died in their 30s from breast cancer, and its chances of being passed on to her female children are very high. Using PGD, all female embryos will be tested for the presence of this gene, and will only be inserted into the uterus if they do not have it. It is similar to the cystic fibrosis illustration except that any female offspring born carrying this gene will be normal (as far as this gene is concerned) for at least 30 years. She will have a normal life, although her life will be overshadowed by the possibility of dying of breast cancer at a young age. Selection here is becoming more ambiguous, since its therapeutic intent has far more of a future orientation. In this sense, it has far less in common with what happens naturally. The selection between embryos is to suit the aspiration of human beings to look for good health for many years to come. But there is no hint of coercion. Is this unacceptable eugenics, or is the term still an inappropriate one?

Scenario 4

In this instance PGD is carried out because the couple in question have three boys and now want a girl. There is no therapeutic intent. They admit that this is a social desire, although they view it as being a legitimate one. Whatever arguments can sometimes be made in favour of social sex selection, this is the closest we have come to eugenics, even though it is a non-coercive form of eugenics. Should arguments against this form of sex selection be framed in terms of eugenics? Normal embryos are being discarded in this case, but they have also been discarded in some of the previous scenarios. Are the intentions of those who wish to move in this direction eugenicist in nature?

Scenario 5

Way into the future it may prove possible to employ PGD to alter genes so that embryos are manipulated and designed to have the biological characteristics we might desire: the blue-eyed, intelligent, tall individuals so beloved of science fiction. We find it difficult, if not impossible, to take such scenarios seriously, but what we have here is positive eugenics in all its glory. Such a scenario is replete with narcissistic desires and humanistic aspirations, and one can object on those grounds. However, from a scientific perspective one can far more readily dismiss these fanciful pictures on account of their lack of scientific integrity. They will not occur in anything like the way they are envisaged. By all means dismiss them as eugenicist, but it is unhelpful to use this as a basis for arguing that PGD inevitably has a eugenicist orientation.

Of these scenarios, number 5 is closest to anything resembling classical eugenics. One could conclude that it is eugenics in what we might call a strong sense, although there is no element of compulsion about it. However, its fanciful nature should exclude it from being considered as anything resembling Nazi-style eugenics. Scenario 4 has similarities, and its eugenic overtones are unmistakable. It is also a present reality, and hence is more problematic than scenario 5.

Scenario 1 cannot be thought of as eugenics on most definitions. Scenario 2, PGD in its standard therapeutic form, is only eugenics in the weakest possible sense. However, in my view, its very positive therapeutic intent surely separates it from even this form of eugenics. Scenario 3 is eugenics of a slightly stronger sort, and without a doubt it raises numerous ethical questions. Its eugenicist overtones complicate what are already very challenging issues.

No matter what conclusions we reach on the eugenicist overtones of these various scenarios, we need to remind ourselves that today's society is distinctly different from that of the beginning of the twentieth century in that there is no state eugenics movement. Rather than a state-mandated system which, in its attempt to prevent the birth of genetically 'undesirable' children, prevents those with undesirable genes from procreating, we have a system that seeks to enable those with a genetic predisposition to certain diseases and disabilities to have children unaffected by those conditions. As a result, contemporary society is not demanding that only those with good genes are allowed to procreate; rather, the opposite. The focus of PGD is to assist those with predispositions to certain devastating illnesses and disabilities to have children, minus those conditions.

But further issues are at stake here, depending upon the character of the state. The conclusions we have reached would not hold if the state mandated that people use PGD. Neither would they if people were compelled to use only embryos with desirable characteristics. The same would apply if the state decreed that it would not support any children born with genetic diseases or disabilities when the parents had refused to use PGD to avoid their birth. In each of these instances, the state would be placing its own interests above those of individuals and families. However, as we have seen, such directions are far from implicit within most applications of PGD as we know them today. Consequently, eugenic considerations come to the fore principally when PGD is applied within a coercive environment.

Of course, it is relatively easy to speculate and imagine worlds far removed from our own, where PGD could be used to implement rampant eugenic aspirations. Often, when PGD comes under debate, parental autonomy is considered to be foundational. But what if an autonomous decision by the parents were to lead to the loss of their child's freedom? While this is mere speculation, one can imagine an embryo created (via PGD) to be intelligent, enabling the parents to have offspring capable of achieving well in life. Or, alternatively, imagine an embryo with the potential for great athletic ability, endowing the family with a future world champion. Coercion is implicit in all these scenarios, and yet even these would probably not differ greatly from current behavioural and environmental routes lacking any hint of genetic selection and modification. Environmental manipulation may be as powerful as genetic manipulation in its potentially devastating effects on children. All such should be condemned.

PGD is a technical means to an end. The nature of the human response is seen in the end to which this technique is put. In no way is this predetermined by the technique. In extreme circumstances PGD could be used for eugenicist goals. But this does not constitute the gist of PGD as we know it today.

Theological Responses

Any particular theological response to PGD tends to parallel views held on the status of human embryos. For those who view embryos as human persons, discarding such embryos in PGD is unacceptable, as is the selection of one embryo over another. For Christians with a gradualist view of an embryo's developing personhood, PGD will probably be seen as acceptable under some circumstances, since it involves a balancing of goods, and takes account of the health and wellbeing of future children and adults. However, even those who view PGD with distaste should not do so on eugenic grounds.

Theological insights would be expected to emphasise the importance of the voluntary nature of a procedure like PGD, and hence should argue against coercion. They would also be expected to call into serious question any ephemeral use of PGD, but to applaud therapeutic goals as long as these do not jeopardise the integrity of human personhood. Striving for health has been an underlying rationale in much Christian-based care, and this would play a prominent role in the use of PGD, in spite of the inevitable ethical challenges posed by the procedure. But we would not expect the allegedly eugenic nature of PGD to feature in theological arguments.

It is important for Christians to examine the reasons why society encourages PGD. Much of this comes from the desire to have healthy children and all that that entails. The problem here is that expectations of health continue to escalate, transforming the notion of health itself. The result is that PGD is being used for an ever increasing range of conditions. This is where PGD becomes questionable, since it is guided by both good and bad motivating factors. We can focus on the burden that the parents will be placed under upon the birth of a child with this or that debilitating condition – including financial burdens. Or, we can discuss the life that this same child will have to endure. Such emphases have to be balanced by an unqualified acceptance of all individuals, no matter what disabilities or diseases they may suffer from. Christians will wish to respond with compassion to all families struggling with these issues.

The balancing of goods is so clearly evident in discussions of PGD. Although I have rejected assertions that PGD is inherently eugenicist, we do need to be constantly reminded that it has overtones of sacrificing the weak in the interests of the strong,[16] and that it can readily assume exploitative connotations. The greed of a materialistic philosophy demonstrated in an ethic of destruction is ever present, as it is in many other biomedical realms. The agonising dilemma presented by PGD is whether it is possible to use it whilst still striving to espouse an ethic of protection, preservation and care. How can this ethic be applied when children and parents are those of concern, alongside embryos? And which of these groups is in greatest need of this ethic of protection? Our responsibility as human beings made in God's image is a mutual and overarching responsibility that has to encompass the power and prospects opened up by PGD. And this is no mean challenge.

16   P. Saunders, 'Deadly Questions. ... On Prenatal Screening', *Nucleus*, October 1998, pp.34–37.

GERARD MANNION

Genetics and the Ethics of Community

In 1998, the World Health Organisation recommended that prenatal diagnosis should only be performed in order to benefit the foetus, as opposed to being carried out to satisfy parental curiosity. Yet, with the advent of new technologies, prenatal diagnosis of many kinds is now being carried out for a wide variety of reasons that, it would appear, might not only supersede the interests of the foetus, but could even work contrary to such interests.[1] And the emergence of technologies that push back such diagnosis even to the pre-implantation stage of the (IVF-produced) embryo has raised a number of pressing questions of an ethical and, in particular, social nature.[2]

Indeed, developments in genetic science and technology are taking place at an incredibly rapid pace, not least of all due to the momentum and excitement generated across the globe by the Human Genome project (HGP). Thankfully, numerous organisations have also been formed to try to ensure that the ethical, legal and social implications of such advances are not overlooked. But, despite their best

---

1   An earlier version of this chapter appeared as 'Genetics and the Ethics of Community', in *The Heythrop Journal* 47, April 2006, pp.226–56. What appears here is an updated and abbreviated version.

2   The United Nations *Declaration on Bioethics*, finally adopted on 19 October 2005, states in 'Human Dignity and Human Rights', article 3, that: 'Human dignity, human rights and fundamental freedoms are to be fully preserved. The interests and welfare of the individual should have priority over the sole interest of science or society.' But the protracted disagreements over this UNESCO declaration, along with the watering down of the force of its earlier drafts, further suggest that much work remains to be done in safeguarding the rights and dignity of both individuals and communities in the face of new developments in biotechnology. Note, further, that there are tensions even within the logic of such a statement designed to promote rights: an individual could demand certain benefits that might be detrimental to others and to society in the long run.

efforts, important elements of the ethical, social and, indeed, legal implications of genetic science frequently continue to be overlooked, even ignored, or at best given cursory attention.

Worse still, decisions in the field of genetics are at times made and presented as if the ethical debates had already been adequately treated and all moral considerations addressed, when the truth is very different. Nor is it always easy or desirable to separate the ethical, legal and social questions posed by new developments. The impact of developments in genetic science upon communities is one field of enquiry that entails each of these areas. This will be illustrated throughout this chapter, the modest aim of which is to raise and discuss certain key issues and to open the debate about them to a wider audience beyond the medical, scientific, legislative and genethics professional 'communities'.[3]

I shall therefore explore the impact of genetics upon communities through focusing, in particular, upon certain developments in reproductive science. After introducing core issues and technologies, the chapter engages with particular ethical concerns in relation to the 'shadow' of eugenics over such developments, and then explores the role of legislative debates and procedures in transforming social attitudes, values and, hence, norms. I then turn to consider debates concerning the 'quality of life ethic' now prevalent in healthcare ethics, and move on to discuss the issue of genetic discrimination – focusing, in particular, upon discrimination against disabled persons, as a representative instance of the actual ethical and social/ communitarian implications of the foregoing. I end by raising questions deemed worthy of further exploration and debate. There is a need to explore the ways in which the ethics of genetics is presently shaped and practised in order to discern better the particular social and communitarian implications of certain technological advances.

---

3   Such matters are very complex, as Ellen Wright Clayton has indicated: 'Understanding the social effects of genomics requires an analysis of the ways in which genetic information and a genetic approach to disease affect people individually, within their families and communities, and in their social and working lives'. See Ellen Wright Clayton, 'Ethical, Legal and Social Implications of Genomic Medicine', *New England Journal of Medicine* 349, 7 August 2003, p.562.

I hope that this chapter will also serve two further purposes in the wider context of the whole volume. First, it will complement the discussions within other chapters, particularly those by Gareth Jones concerning PGD itself, as well as his other contributions on the human body, enhancement and regulatory procedures. Secondly, I hope that it might serve as an illustration of that type of theologically-informed ethics that I talked about in my own earlier chapter.

I hope, too, that the fruitfulness of a dialogical bridge between the different disciplines will also be further illustrated; this chapter addresses the situation in societies such as the UK, Europe and the United States. The ethical discourse is explicit. My theological back-drop is more implicit, yet permeates each and every page. Hence the notion of community itself; of human persons as inherently social beings; the inherent dignity and worth of all persons; the necessity of speaking out for the concerns of the neglected and marginalised, the apparent 'least' within society; the need for greater inclusivity and acceptance of all; the fact that we all have numerous social resp-onsibilities as well as rights – indeed the fundamental principle of Christian social ethics in general: all inform and are somehow utilised and reflected in this paper. Some might ask why they are not explicitly couched here in theological language and terminology – such could easily be provided. But then the chapter would cease to illustrate that theologically-*informed* ethics can make positive and constructive contributions to scientific, medical and legislative debates in secular and pluralist societies; that one need not be familiar with nor even convinced of the theological beliefs and moral traditions that inform the argument herein in order to gain something from the resultant moral discernment.

To explain a little further: implicit Christian theological values are at work here, shaping and informing what follows, and yet the chapter can be heard, and identified with, by numerous non-Christian communities and individuals alike. Values of core importance to the Christian moral traditions can also offer hope and resources for ethical discernment to a wider, more pluralistic and secular society. Indeed one might find out just how many values are actually shared across and between different religious and secular worldviews and value systems. I do not hide from the fact that the ethical discernment contained herein is theologically-informed; nor do I in any way apologise for this.

One further introductory remark is of importance. In this chapter, I am critical of some scientific, medical and legislative practices. But it is not at all my intention to over-generalise in a negative way about scientists, medical practitioners or legislators, nor do I seek to deny that there are a great many people working in such fields who are acutely aware of the expertise pertaining in the ethical debates concerned. Indeed, I indicate here at the outset (and this volume helps to illustrate on a wider basis) just how engaged with the ethics of genetics many people across these fields actually are.

Setting the Social Scene: From Cinematic Thought-Experiment to Contemporary Debates

In the film, *Gattaca*, set 'in the not too distant future', Ethan Hawke plays a 'faith birth' – a child whose parents had opted not to undergo the (by then) more usual process of having a geneticist screen several of their fertilised embryos to determine the most 'superior specimen' to implant in the mother's womb. But even the church-linked hospital where he is born avails itself of some of the latest technology and so, soon after his delivery, the 'life-map', the fate if you like, of Hawke's character, Vincent, is revealed in a printout following a simple blood test. He has a high percentage likelihood of developing several debilitating conditions, including a neurological problem, attention deficit disorder and manic depression. But the most worrying revelation of all is that he has a heart condition which will almost certainly, it is pronounced, prove fatal and lead to his premature death at about the age of 30.

His parents soon discover the trials and tribulations of having such a 'handicapped' child. For example, schools turn him away in case he might have an accident, their reason being that their insurance policy would not cover any liability for him. The parents thus resolve, when contemplating having a second child, not to make the same 'mistake' again, and they turn to a geneticist to 'weed out' particular diseases and imperfections for this next child. In other words, they have a number of embryos screened and choose the 'best' to implant into the mother.

Such genetically selected, engineered and, in the eyes of their society, 'superior' embryos (and hence superior children) have fast become the preferred choice for parents of a certain class and privilege. Poor Vincent is left to join the new underclass of inferior human beings with inherent 'defects'. They are left only to occupy menial and low-paid jobs. In that society, where random genetic tests reveal not simply one's true identity, one's genetic 'fingerprint', but also the current state and future development of one's health, the opportunities for those who have any such 'defects' are extremely limited. They become known as 'de-*gene*rates' and their legal status is as 'in-valids'. And those whose parents chose the 'best' embryos, with the bare minimum of imperfections, become the high-flyers, destined for the top careers and most amenable lifestyles.

But it is not simply those whose likely imperfections are known before birth who suffer the fate of the 'degenerates'. Those who fall foul of misfortune later in life are soon excluded from the best careers and life opportunities as well, as Jude Law's character, Jerome Morrow, finds out when he is disabled following a road accident. When social values and norms are transformed, all members of that society are obviously thus affected.

I shall not spoil the plot for those who have yet to see this excellent film, but *Gattaca* is a story of the triumph of human resilience over prejudice and discrimination, and also over the technologisation of society. It is the story of one 'degenerate' who simply refuses to accept the hand (and so life) that society tells him fate has dealt him. It is, of course, no exaggeration to say that the reproductive technology witnessed in *Gattaca* is, in many ways, ever more becoming science reality rather than science fiction. The technology for prenatal embryonic screening is already available; and the name for this technique is pre-implantation genetic diagnosis (PGD).[4] Gareth Jones has outlined this technique in much greater detail elsewhere in this volume, so here I shall presume that my readers have already acquainted themselves with his text.

The UK Human Fertilisation and Embryology Authority (HFEA) defines the technique in this way: 'Pre-implantation genetic diagnosis (PGD) involves the removal of a cell from an embryo created by *in vitro* fertilisation. The cell is then tested to see if the embryo carries a genetic disorder. This is usually three days after fertilisation when the embryo has six to ten cells.' And elsewhere: '[PGD] is a technique which involves the genetic testing of embryos created *in vitro* for deleterious, heritable genetic conditions which are known to be present in the family of those seeking treatment and from which the embryos are known to be at risk.'[5] A further technique sometimes carried out following PGD is 'Human Leukocyte Antigen (HLA) tissue typing [which] is an additional step to determine the tissue-compatibility of embryos free from the disorder with an existing sibling'. This latter technique was outlawed in December 2002 – a legal finding which 'disappointed' the HFEA, whose appeal against it proved successful in April 2003. The HLA techniques permitted were extended by the HFEA in July 2004, when the HFEA ensured that Britain became the first country to allow screening for 'therapeutic' purposes (for example, to allow a sibling to be born with the necessary genetic material to help an existing child), as opposed to the previous situation when screening was restricted to that carried out to detect

4   For a clear and concise introductory discussion of the technique of PGD see
     Norman Ford, *The Prenatal Person: Ethics from Conception to Birth* (Oxford:
     Blackwell, 2002), pp.61–62, p.73. See also: A. M. Nagy et al., 'Scientific and
     Ethical Issues of Preimplantation Diagnosis', *Annals of Medicine* 30, 1998,
     pp.1–6; Bonnie Steinbeck, 'Preimplantation Genetic Diagnosis and Embryo
     Selection', in Justine Burley and John Harris, *A Companion to Genethics*
     (Oxford: Blackwell, 2004), pp.175–90. For wider debates in this area, beyond
     PGD, see Bonnie Steinbeck, *Life Before Birth: The Moral and Legal Status of
     Embryos and Newborns* (New York: OUP, 1997); Richard A. McCormick,
     'Who or What is the Pre-embryo', chapter 4 of his *Corrective Vision* (London:
     Sheed and Ward, 1994).
5   HFEA's working definition can be found on their website: www.hfea.gov.uk/
     AboutHFEA/HFEAPolicy/Preimplantationgeneticdiagnosis.

potential diseases. The HFEA proceeded to state that it would make a 'case by case' and 'condition by condition' decision on whether to allow PGD, only as and when the technique for screening for each condition becomes available.

But it should here be noted that genes relating to an increased likelihood of developing diseases can still only be screened for in a very few cases. Even then, such knowledge is often of very limited value. But the impact upon individuals, their families and society in general can be enormous. Even in the case of those individuals who have an extremely small chance of carrying such genes, the pressure to test is enormous once screening is an option. This poses a whole range of moral dilemmas. For example, whether to tell relatives (who may then also feel obliged to be tested), or employers (in the USA there have been instances of individuals losing their jobs after doing so), or insurance companies (healthcare benefits may be, and have been, withdrawn if one does so – even if the policy was taken out years before screening took place).

At the moment, it is still uncertain to what extent many societies will opt for either permissive or more restrictive legislation in the application of PGD. It would appear that many societies are moving more towards the former, but, as on many such issues, opinion is deeply divided both within and across national boundaries. Even aside from embryonic screening, we do, of course, have much more widely available forms of prenatal screening, which can already detect and reveal much about the present and future health of a foetus.

What *Gattaca* helps to illustrate is that as technology advances, particularly when that technology is applied to healthcare and its provision, social attitudes too are transformed and, in turn, so is community life. Yet too much ethical debate about genetics focuses primarily upon the individual. In 2002, the report of the US-based Hastings Center included an article which stated that:

> In recent years there has been increasing attention devoted to the possibility that genetic research can harm communities. The risk of group discrimination and the difficult task of obtaining informed consent at the level of the

community rather than the individual have posed challenges for scientists doing population genetics, pharmocogenomic, and related research.[6]

And it is not simply particular common interest groups that are at risk (for example, those who share a particular disability or condition). There are dangers posed by such technology to the flourishing of community in general. Although a full consideration of all the ways in which the Human Genome project and genetic science pose a threat to communities, and to communitarian rights, norms and values, is beyond the scope of a single chapter, we can come to appreciate some of the fundamental issues involved through focusing upon particular (and representative) examples of social and communitarian implications of the genetic revolution.[7] So we are thus concerned with social ontologies,[8] and the ethics of community is here understood to involve an examination of the role played by various (and sometimes competing) social ontologies.

For those concerned about what is here meant by the term 'community', I am inclined to say that to seek a rigid definition is almost the same as committing the naturalistic fallacy when asking for a rigid definition of the term 'good'. However, because the term is a contested one, some indication of what I take a community to be is

6   Holly C. Goodin, Benjamin Wilfond, Karina Boehm, and Barbara Bowles
     Biesecker, 'Unintended Messages: The Ethics of Teaching Genetic Dilemmas',
     Hastings Center Report 32, 2002, p.37.
7   Thus, for example, further questions relating to population genetics, related
     issues concerning individual, familial and communitarian consent or the
     implications of initiatives such as the HapMap Project which aims to develop a
     public resource that will help researchers find genes associated with human
     disease and response to pharmaceuticals (in relation to which latter, see
     www.hapmap.org).
8   The term *social ontology* shall be understood as a conception, which can also
     be developed into a hermeneutical framework of, or at least some general and
     multifaceted understanding of, human social existence. So, a social ontology is,
     as the name suggests, an understanding of collective, social, human *being* (and
     a preference in favour of such an understanding prevailing in our various moral,
     political, legislative and even scientific debates); and is *social* as opposed to
     any ontology that gives primacy to the individual, (cf. the citation below from
     Moltmann). Conceptions of community are a form of social ontology. Particular social ontologies inform the practices associated with community.

necessary. At a fundamental level, it is being-in-relation, an acknowledgement of the interconnectedness of human existence. Community
involves an attempt to live in awareness of the fact that reality is so
interconnected.[9] Consider Judith Merkle's explanation:

> Community is a center of multi-layered interactions among people. These
> traditions and rituals are preserved and developed. Life skills are learned and
> called forth. Discipline is nurtured and expected. Fidelity and accountability to
> the community are practised. At best community is a way of life that shapes
> and defines members' identity. True community shows itself in alliance for a
> common cause, a life beyond itself. Community is also a moral stance. The
> parable of the Good Samaritan (Luke 10:25-37) defines a neighbor or a
> community in terms of compassionate behavior.[10]

Reality is hence understood as being community oriented.[11] Hence by
the phrase 'ethics of community' I simply mean a concern with the
moral issues pertaining to, and a commitment to the advancement of,

9   Here, the words of Jürgen Moltmann are instructive: '[A] *person* is not an
      individual. The distinction is simple, but seldom made. According to its Latin
      meaning, an *individuum* is something ultimately indivisible, like "atom" in
      Greek. A person, in comparison, is – as Martin Buber showed (following
      Hegel, Feuerbach, and Hölderlin) – the individual human being in the resonant
      field of his or her relationships, the relationships of I, Thou and We, I-Myself
      and I-It. In the network of relationships, the person becomes the human subject
      of taking and giving, listening and doing, experiencing and touching, hearing
      and responding. We approach humanism only when we pass from
      individualism to personalism', Jürgen Moltmann, 'Freedom in Community
      between Globalization and Individualism: Market Value and Human Dignity',
      in Jürgen Moltmann, *God for a Secular Society: The Public Relevance of
      Theology* (London: SCM, 1999), p.156.
10   Judith A. Merkle, *From the Heart of the Church: The Catholic Social Tradition*
      (Collegeville: Michael Glazier, 2004), p.243.
11   Although I prefer primacy being given to ontological, as opposed to functional,
      understandings of community, I nonetheless warm very much to Merkle's
      interpretation of community. Indeed, in its outworking, Merkle's understanding
      actually combines both functional and ontological aspects, and is obviously
      replete with ontological implications.

the lives of human social beings; that is, in particular, of communities.[12] Let us discern some initial questions for consideration.

We begin by noting that the threat posed to our social existence is not something that has first visited humanity in the twenty-first century – social engineering based upon so-called advances in science and medicine has haunted numerous communities and societies before. I refer to eugenics, which may not have altogether disappeared earlier in the twentieth century as conclusively as some believe. Many who advance the cause of certain developments in science do so because they subscribe to very particular (and often hierarchical) conceptions of social reality. So, our first issue to be considered follows.

Eugenics and the Transformation of Social Values and Norms

Various studies have demonstrated that behind much of the research, funding and justification for genetic and later genomic research lie causal factors that were initially set in train by those actively engaged in the theory and practice of eugenics.[13] The connection is far from

12   Of course, the term, as used here, is meant in the sense of relating *an* ethics of community to ethical considerations in genetic science and medicine, as opposed to suggesting there is only one ethics of community or of genetics. To help give some hint towards the argument that I shall develop, consider the following words from Frank Kirkpatrick: 'Mutual community is the singular locus that creates and reconciles diversity, particularity, fulfilment, and universality; the conditions of human community set the limits to diversity but at the same time provide the basis for its expression since no community can be fulfilling to its members unless it nourishes their particularities as individuals', Frank G. Kirkpatrick, *A Moral Ontology for a Theistic Ethic: Gathering The Nations in Love and Justice* (Harmondsworth, Ashgate, 2003), p.6.

13   Obviously genetic theories preceded the development of eugenics itself. But today eugenics refers to a more particular branch of science than such earlier theories and is hence employed in the contemporary sense. Distinctions are made between negative eugenics and positive eugenics – here I refer to what is termed negative eugenics.

fanciful. After all, eugenics is defined in the *OED* as the 'science of improving the population by control of inherited qualities'. So, many of the figures involved had an agenda aimed towards social engineering.[14] Of course, many of the more prominent theorists in the field of eugenics were forced to change their terminology and justificatory arguments in the wake of the revelations concerning the Nazi eugenics programme. Hence, in other words, the previously much more widespread and popular field of 'eugenics' became transformed into 'genetics',[15] so as to avoid association with the particular application of eugenics carried out by the Nazi regime. But many such theorists did *not* change their fundamental views or ultimate aims.[16]

So why should we be concerned today? Because in the present climate what, for some, may constitute the 'unthinkable' need not necessarily remain as such in the eyes of the wider society. Attitudes change and with them, in turn, social norms. Technology may presently be running far ahead of the ethical debates once again, and the spectre of eugenics is one of the most challenging aspects of the genetic revolution which communities must face. The point is that

14   Cf. D. B. Paul, *Controlling Human Heredity: 1865 to the Present* (Amherst, NY: Humanity Books, 1998), especially chapter 7, 'From Eugenics to Human Genetics'. See also: 'Eugenics and Its Shadow', chapter 2 of Allen Buchanan, Dan W. Brock, Norman Daniels and Daniel Wikler, *From Chance to Choice: Genetics and Justice* (Cambridge: Cambridge University Press, 2000). A chapter by Celia Deane-Drummond also provides an informative discussion of the ethical issues involved here: 'Living in the Shadow of Eugenics', in *Genetics and Christian Ethics* (Cambridge: Cambridge University Press, 2005).

15   As D. B. Paul has illustrated, 'The connection between eugenics and human genetics' is somewhat striking, as witnessed in the history and development of the American Society of Human Genetics, founded in 1948. Paul states that: 'From the start, human genetics was intertwined with – and sometimes indistinguishable from – eugenics', *Controlling Human Heredity*, p.121. A further point worthy of sustained reflection is that the US journal, *Eugenics Quarterly*, changed its name to *Social Biology* in 1968, ibid., p.125.

16   For example, the profession of 'genetic counselling', now so widespread in the United States, was initially encouraged, resourced and developed by those advocates of eugenics as a means to encourage reproductive practices which would further their social engineering agenda. (Hence it was a very directive practice in its original incarnation, as opposed to today's – supposed – non-directional norm.)

174 Gerard Mannion

scientific developments are transforming attitudes in a wide variety of forms, with a broad range of implications.

Much of the evidence currently available in such areas, along with the discussions in the field, would suggest that many particular communities and other social groupings are at risk from greater discrimination as a result of advances in genetic research,[17] alongside the pursuit of the scientific, medical, economic and political benefits which might accrue from the Human Genome project. And the effect upon particular communities has an effect, in turn, upon the wider society and community in general. Attitudes can be transformed and/or accentuated by genetic theories and technological developments, and often for a wide variety of reasons. Whether intentional or not, scientific developments can provide support to unpalatable social attitudes and transformed social norms. Of course, sometimes the science is misrepresented or its claims exaggerated – but this is not infrequently done with the assistance of members of the scientific professions themselves. Witness the range of claims made for the societal 'benefits' that eugenics would bring about, and compare this with some of the media stories concerning recent developments in reproductive genetics.

In particular, when economic expediency becomes the prime concern of those in power, the greater is the risk of discrimination against certain groups. As D. B. Paul has argued, if history teaches us anything in relation to the issues surrounding eugenics, it is that:

> when motives are mixed, financial considerations tend over time to displace other values. … [W]hat may be unthinkable when times are flush may come to seem only good common sense when they are not. In the 1920s most geneticists

17 Various examples are discussed in the literature concerning the risk of discrimination: existing risks are posed to groups of persons who share the same or similar condition or disability, along with their families, loved ones and others closely involved in their lives. *Potential* risks are posed to communities formed through race, particularly those who, again, are susceptible to particular conditions; to those with particular addictions; those susceptible to committing crime; to those deemed to be of limited intelligence and/or education; to those who share, for example, homosexual orientation. Even those of particular social classes are at potential risk from new or renewed forms of discrimination.

found the idea of compulsory sterilization repugnant. In the midst of the Depression they no longer did.[18]

Paul provides a wealth of evidence, as well as a broad survey of the changing developments in social attitudes towards eugenics and genetic research and technology, to support her argument that the history of eugenics is one of 'diverse motivations'.[19] How is all this relevant to our present-day situation? It is because it illustrates that changing economic and political factors can swiftly transform what may be generally considered simply as unpalatable and ethically uninformed scientific beliefs and developments into social realities with profoundly unethical consequences. Again; changing perceptions can lead to transformed social norms and values. Whilst such transformations can sometimes be beneficial, for instance the nineteenth-century shift in many societies towards perceiving the provision of universal education as a societal obligation, they can also be deeply disturbing. In our present times the reality is that new and renewed forms of discrimination (against both individuals and communities) are already becoming part of the fabric of many societies.

Further, Paul believes that important lessons can be drawn from the story of eugenics, which can inform our discussions on genetic research and medicine today:

> As a story of destructive state power, the history of eugenics teaches us one lesson. As a story of attitudes toward people with disabilities, it teaches another. The first reinforces the view that reproduction should be a private affair. The second leads us to reflect on attitudes toward the disabled, those whom Margaret Sanger as well as Adolf Hitler thought 'should never have been born'. In this second story, acts are not benign simply because their agents are private citizens. Indeed, if we insist on absolute reproductive autonomy we must accept the use of genetic technologies to prevent the birth of those who are unwanted for any reason: that they will be the 'wrong' gender, or sexual orientation, or of short stature, or prone to obesity, or ... [When] used this way, medical genetics will surely reinforce a host of social prejudices.[20]

18   D. B. Paul, *Controlling Human Heredity*, p.134.
19   Ibid.
20   Ibid., p.135.

None of the foregoing is sensationalism or unwarranted scandalising and, indeed, evidence is accumulating which proves such suspicions to be well founded. Indeed, we may witness a scenario coming to pass in which state power and private prejudice combine to build an alliance whereby genuine reproductive autonomy is, in effect, eroded and manipulated to serve the vested interests of state and corporate bodies. An instance of this is where pressure is put upon couples to undergo prenatal or pre-implantation diagnosis, and where abortion of 'defective' foetuses or destruction of 'defective' embryos is then presented as the only rational response. Another example is that of some states in the US employing such tactics in the light of their budgeting limits for the provision of services to disabled persons and people with debilitating medical conditions.

Thus, there are some members of societies and communities who have disabilities and are now suffering renewed prejudice, as well as new *forms* of prejudice, and this is not simply at the hands of the ignorant, malicious or ill-informed.[21] Sophisticated philosophical ethicists, medical practitioners, scientific researchers and public policy makers have proved to be quite capable of misunderstanding and ignorance, as well as of prejudice and discrimination, on such matters.

I have suggested that genetics today is prone to being used for purposes of social engineering and that the resultant discrimination against both individuals and communities is a very real problem demanding ethical attention.[22] But what facilitates such a situation

21   The literature on genetic prejudice and discrimination is already large and growing. See, for example, Lisa N. Geller, 'Current Developments in Genetic Discrimination', chapter 13 of *The Double-Edged Helix: Social Implications of Genetics in a Diverse Society*, ed. J. S. Alper et al. (Baltimore: Johns Hopkins University Press, 2002); see also essays on various debates of relevance here in Justine Burley and John Harris, *A Companion to Genethics* (Oxford, Blackwell, 2004), Parts IV and V.

22   For examples of other representative views concerning the relationships of PGD to eugenics, see J. Milliez and C. Sureau, 'Pre-implantation Diagnosis and the Eugenics Debate: Our Responsibilities to Future Generations', in *Ethical Dilemmas in Assisted Reproduction*, ed. F. Shenfield and C. Sureau (New York: Parthenon Publishing Group, 1997); Joseph D. Schulman and R. G. Edwards, 'Preimplantation Diagnosis is Disease Control Not Eugenics', *Human Reproduction* 11, 1996, pp.463–64.

coming to pass? Whence do these new social norms and values of concern emerge? One area worthy of exploration is the nature of the legislative process in genetic science and medicine and the effect that this has upon the transformation of social values.

In Part Three of this volume the topics of legislation and regulation are explored in greater detail; so here let me make but a few observations relevant to the concerns of those later chapters. Societal opinions, beliefs, and hence norms, are continuously being transformed by developments in genetic science. Thus, social ontologies, in turn, are transformed. And such developments are not always unintended consequences of changing technological paradigms. Just as in other areas of life, we need to become more aware, with regard to ethics, of how governments and scientists are extremely effective in manipulating the media and public opinion.

Further Recent Developments

There have been numerous further developments since an earlier version of the text of this chapter was published, and each and every one of these developments serves to further highlight the need for greater ethical consideration and debate to be facilitated in relation to such technological innovations and their regulation. Ten years on from the famous cloning of Dolly the Sheep, the year 2006 was a very busy one for scientists and legislators concerned with these and related technologies, and hence also for ethicists engaged with these issues. The potential progress trumpeted in the aftermath of Dolly's cloning has, however, been considerably less rapid than might have been anticipated.

Let us survey a sample of some of the main developments in recent times. Several such developments took place in the UK, entailing yet further relaxation in the regulation of what research in these fields is permitted and what is not. There has been further liberalisation, on the part of the HFEA, of the regulations governing which medical conditions can be tested for using PGD, and steps have been taken to allow women to receive 'half-price' IVF treatment if they 'donate' some of their own eggs to be used by scientists in research. Indeed, such moves towards financial remuneration for donors followed the 2005 HFEA ruling that opened the way for children born as a result of donated embryos and gametes to learn the identity of the donors in later life, should they wish to do so. France's ethical commission has been exploring similar issues. Thus it is not simply an increasing liberalisation of regulation that we are witnessing here; we are equally witnessing an increasing commodification of human reproduction itself. Cases of trafficking in oocytes (eggs), embryos, and gametes alike, along with their importation into countries with more liberal regulations in research and reproductive technology, have emerged on a growing scale. In March 2005, the European Parliament passed a resolution against trading in eggs and also identified the need for egg donations to be more strictly regulated. Romania, in particular, appeared to be one country in Europe where illegal practices had been commonly taking place, with many of the products of such activity finding their way to the UK.

More and more countries began to examine how and why they might relax their restrictions on embryonic stem cell research, including many parts of the USA. But, in that country, the debate still rages on, illustrated most vividly by the fact that the US President, in September 2006, exercised a veto to prevent a liberalising bill on this issue – allowing public funds to support such research – from becoming federal law, despite the Senate following the lead of the House of Representatives and passing the bill. The majority in both houses was not sufficient to override the presidential veto. Even the President's own Republican party is deeply divided on the issue. At the other side of the globe, Singapore's parliament passed permissive legislation in September 2004. Across Europe, similar debates were taking place, particularly in France, where an official report recommended embryonic stem cell research, along with permitting therapeutic cloning too. The Biomedicines agency in France thus began to grant licences for such research in 2006. Nonetheless, earlier in the same year, the chair of France's National Ethical Advisory Committee (CCNE), Didier Sicard, spoke out against France's increasing obsession with prenatal screening and the impact this was having upon the disabled, and on French society's perception of what constitutes a 'normal' child.[23]

Indeed, such issues divided Europe generally, and its legislature went through a series of protracted debates and votes in both 2005 and 2006 in relation to these technologies. Eventually, following discussions in June and July of the same year, the European Union, by a narrow majority, also authorised the use of Union funds to finance research involving adult and embryonic stem cells. The decision, awaiting later ratification in the European Parliament, was clarified in a compromise by the Council of Ministers – allowing research on stem cell lines produced elsewhere, but forbidding the destruction of embryos following extraction of cells involved in any Union-funded research, and also prohibiting reproductive cloning.

Israel recently changed its law on foetal sex selection. Once only permitted on medical grounds, families with four or more children of one sex may now 'choose' whether to proceed with the pregnancy of a particular child. Also in 2006, one research group, the Advanced Cell Technology team, based in Massachusetts and led by Professor Robert Lanza, claimed to be able to create, using PGD technology, embryonic stem cells without destroying the embryos involved. Although the journal *Nature* ran with the findings, their validity and reliability were quickly challenged. The work of the South Korean researcher, Hwang Woo-Suk, who claimed to have obtained stem cell lines via cloning, came under increasing scrutiny and was regarded with growing scepticism. Some of his research was found to be fraudulent and the paper announcing such results was withdrawn. This was followed by further censure from the South Korean authorities and by the international scientific community generally. (Gareth Jones has, of course, discussed this case, and the wider general issues it illustrates, in more detail in an earlier chapter.) The case certainly demonstrates that the stakes are high in the race to harness such technologies and so to gain the enormous funding and subsequent financial benefits that many believe might be the fruit of such work.

By 2007, the UK would allow PGD for diseases which might only possibly develop, as opposed to being highly likely or certain to

23   *Le Croix*, 3 March 2006.

develop. A private clinic in London used PGD to remove embryos with genes that would predispose the child to the risk of developing a squint, and a public hospital, the *Eastman*, used PGD to 'weed out' embryos with genes linked to susceptibility to developing certain types of breast cancer. The UK even permitted screening for diseases, such as Alzheimer's, that could not possibly develop in the subject until much later in life (if, that is, the susceptibility to the gene in question were to be actually passed on at all).[24] Thus, to date, something like fifty conditions in total are tested for in the UK, and about thirty in France; but in the US, where private funding obviously generates interest in, and demand for, a much wider range of possibilities for screening, reports state that the number of conditions for which one might be offered screening runs into hundreds.

The debate on whether adult stem cells and other alternatives would prove actually to be more effective, as well as being obviously more ethically acceptable to most countries, nonetheless continues apace. For example, scientists also hold out the possibility of using stem cells harvested from umbilical cords as an alternative to embryonic manipulation.

Whilst some scientists from around the world have claimed various 'improvements' in animals treated with stem cells, the progress on research which will actually prove of benefit to human beings moves forward at a much slower pace.

What do all these developments mean, beyond the frenzy that reproductive and other genetic technologies are creating in the world of today? Of course, much of the foregoing concerns *potential* risks and a wide variety of contributory factors that require further analysis and discussion. What all such developments appear to point towards is a changing legislative and ethical landscape. But is there any one particular transformation in our social values, and hence our social ontologies, which can be singled out as being particularly worthy of analysis and discussion with regard to the general concerns of this

---

24   Recent developments were discussed in the French daily, *Libération*, 6 November 2007, and were also carried in the *Genethique* press review, 11 November 2007.

chapter? I believe that there is, and a consideration of it can be most illuminating to our debates.

Genetics and the 'Quality of Life'

So, all of the foregoing developments impact upon the nature and wellbeing of our communities, smaller social groupings and other communities within or in proximity to them. So, too, do they impact upon our understanding of what it means to flourish as human beings, both individually and communally. Thus we may state that the boundaries and 'membership' criteria of communities and societies are undergoing change and revision as a result of these developments in genetic science. The 'perfection mindedness' which appears now to be prevailing poses a threat to anyone who falls short of the template for the 'desirable citizen' that influences scientific and legislative debates in many societies.

And, I suggest, this is part of a wider debate and fundamental shift in ethical thinking, influenced and articulated by the work of the applied philosopher Peter Singer. This paradigm shift has been from examining ethical questions from a perspective where all life is viewed as inviolable or *sacred* (and hence the 'sanctity of life' takes precedence) to a situation where the supposed, anticipated, perceived or even actual 'quality' of the life in question prevails.[25] There are consequences of this shift, in the form of transformed social values, norms and ontologies, and the subsequent impact of such axiological transformation upon communities.

One of the primary results of this shift in emphasis is that highly subjective criteria (such as 'quality of life') are now being applied to determine, or at least influence, who can and should be members of our communities and societies, and also to influence decisions about what healthcare benefits certain persons should receive. I make this

---

25 Cf. Peter Singer, 'Is the Sanctity of Life Ethic Terminally Ill?', *Bioethics* 9, 1995, pp.327–43.

statement notwithstanding the prevalence of literature in favour of attempts to offer supposedly objective bases to assess the 'quality of life' for particular individuals or of a population in general, for example the so-called QALYs and DALYs,[26] because there is just as significant a body of literature which challenges the validity of the supposed objectivity of such bases.

So, if it is granted (as so much of this latter literature suggests) that the criteria employed in assessing 'quality of life' are frequently much more subjective than is claimed for them, we now see that, in spite of this, such criteria are even being applied to those who are not yet born and, furthermore (as we have seen), the technology is already available whereby such criteria can be applied to (and their con-sequences implemented upon) those who are yet to be conceived or implanted in the womb.

Let us consider one pertinent example. The renowned ethicist and moral philosopher, Ronald Green, states unequivocally that we have a *moral* obligation 'not to harm' our children 'genetically'. What does he mean by this? In short, that if the technology exists for pre-natal screening to identify the likelihood, or indeed certainty, of an unborn child (or embryo) having a particularly debilitating disease or disability, then it is the moral duty of the parents *not* to bring that child into the world, because to do so would inflict severe suffering upon that child. In a now seminal article, Green recognises that there will be a social impact of such reasoning:

> … the increasing number of diagnosable genetic disorders, including some for which early detection may have therapeutic value, has raised the question

---

26   These denote, respectively, Quality Adjusted Life Years and Disability Adj-usted Life Years. Both involve the assignation of numerical 'scores' pertaining to different conditions and their impact upon the lives of individuals or of populations. The former is, in essence, a form of cost-utility analysis of health intervention; that is, the benefit of healthcare intervention is determined by calculating how many QALYs any person would gain with and without such intervention. DALYs, adopted by the World Bank in 1993, are, on the other hand, supposed to offer a measurement of the 'burden of disease'. This measure goes from a starting point of zero (meaning 'no significant health problem') to a score of 1 (meaning 'death or equivalent').

whether pressure should be brought to bear on parents (or prospective parents) to undergo testing to prevent serious harms to their offspring or society.[27]

But here we must not overlook some of the other communitarian implications of the new technology. Indeed, one might also wish to raise the perhaps unforeseen social implications that can arise from the methodology adopted by Green and many others in their ethical analysis of such dilemmas. Let us consider an example. Although Green usually tends towards the defence of individual reproductive autonomy, he puts forth a detailed argument that 'parents can wrong their children by knowingly or carelessly bringing them into being in certain circumstances of life'.[28] His reasoning is informed by his belief that:

> ... parents are properly regarded as proxy decision-makers for their child's health status ...[29]

He goes on to conclude that:

27 Ronald M. Green, 'Parental Autonomy and the Obligation Not to Harm One's Child Genetically', *Journal of Law, Medicine & Ethics* 25, 1997, p.5.

28 Ibid., p.7. The *functional* nature of Green's reasoning poses further questions, as do the ontological aspects of his statements here and elsewhere (which might well be in danger of being over simplistic). Some might at this point suggest that the Catholic church could be said to be in agreement with this statement in that it permits family planning in circumstances where the birth of a further child would be detrimental to the existing family, but the obvious rejoinder to such a claim is that here we are not concerned with contraception but with genetic screening of existing embryos and foetuses.

29 Green thus appears to equate this situation with, for example, that of a pregnant woman smoking heavily and thus harming her unborn child. His opponents would obviously disagree with his reasoning as to the moral equivalence of such cases. A useful analogy here would be to the different types of euthanasia (such as voluntary contrasted with involuntary and active contrasted with passive). Or again, various interpretations of the principle of double effect are obviously of relevance, particularly the debates surrounding the proportionalist view in relation to natural law thinking (cf. Bernard Hoose, *Proportionalism: The American Debate and its European Roots* (Washington DC: Georgetown University Press, 1987)).

... it is therefore reasonable for a child to feel wronged when poor decision making by parents (or by those who advise them) leads the child to be born with serious impairments or suffering relative to others in its birth cohort.[30]

Now Green identifies himself with a school of ethical theory known as 'omni-impartial public rule morality', in the Rawlsian tradition. But the problem here is a familiar one, namely that many who assume they are exercising value-neutrality and morally-informed rationality are seemingly oblivious to the fact that much of their thinking and argumentation is actually *subjectively* determined, arbitrary and far from being value-neutral. Indeed, to my mind, ethics is not about seeking value-neutrality.[31] It is rather about the opposite state of affairs – the *prevailing* of certain values, and the decisions concerning which values should prevail and which should not – as well as being about the 'implementation' or 'facilitation' of such values being determined on as objective a basis as is humanly possible. Furthermore, I do not believe that the 'quality' of an individual's life, however measured or evaluated, is something that can ever be considered in isolation from their social setting.

Let us now draw together our considerations thus far in relation to debates in the specific area of reproductive technology that we introduced at the beginning of the chapter.

30   Green, 'Parental Autonomy and the Obligation Not to Harm One's Child Genetically', p.8. Green agrees with those who believe misrepresentation law is the correct area of legislation in relation to which such cases should be examined. This appears to overlook the hypothetical point that, on such reasoning (so a case could be made), an aborted foetus could have the 'parents' sued on its behalf – although I here leave aside Green's further questionable arguments as to why 'no one is wronged by *not* being given the opportunity to be born', ibid, p.9.

31   Green allows himself one 'departure' from value-neutrality in the extreme example of one case study (p.13), but appears to believe that such exceptions should be few and far between. And yet Green has actually been far from value-neutral in each case that he discusses here. On a related note, consider the developments pertaining to the French 'Kouchner Law' or 'anti-Perruche' law passed on 4 March 2002, which prohibits anyone from claiming compensation for 'being born' and only allows parents 'non-pecuniary damages'.

Socio-Ethical Implications of Genetic Diagnosis and Screening

Norman Ford offers a concise summary of key moral issues pertaining to pre-implantation genetic screening:

> The use of PGD is linked to the discarding of affected embryos. Many believe that PGD is ethically acceptable. Some hold that in justice there is an ethical duty to prevent defective embryos becoming persons, since they would have to endure lives not worth living. They hold [that] pro-life advocates need to justify their stand in view of the suffering that they indirectly cause in practice. Others believe the decision is a matter for parental autonomy. These positions are consistent with the ethical view that embryos are not persons nor human subjects with an absolute right to life.[32]

Ford also summarises the issues for those who wish to protect life from the moment of conception as follows:

> The deliberate discarding of human embryos at any stage is unethical: bad actions may not be done to prevent suffering. Human embryos should not be subjected to unjust discrimination as if only embryos free of genetic defects are worthy to be born alive.[33]

But here I would add that even if one does not perceive the embryo to be a person, the ethical implications of PGD are no less momentous. For the social and communitarian impact upon *existing* persons is still potentially great. If, for example, society is gradually coming round to the opinion that certain conditions, diseases and disabilities are such that it is preferable that an embryo likely to become a (postnatal) person with any such condition is best destroyed, then this may have

---

32   Norman F. Ford, *The Prenatal Person*, p.73. Ford cites further examples of those who would adopt a similar position to Green here, including Walter Glannon, 'Genes, Embryos and Future People', *Bioethics* 12, 1998, pp.187–205, 209–10; Sozos J. Fasouliotis and Joseph G. Schenker, 'Preimplantation Genetic Diagnostic Principles and Ethics', *Human Reproduction* 13, 1998, p.2241.

33   Ford, *The Prenatal Person*, p.73.

grave consequences for those people who are already in existence and living with such conditions.

So, in relation to prenatal screening and the pressures brought to bear upon prospective parents or, indeed, by them in certain cases (for example where they wish to choose particular characteristics and/or disabilities in their children, or to reject children who would have particular characteristics),[34] we see that the potential threats posed to particular communities, as well as to the very notion of community itself, are indeed serious, unless ethical concerns are brought to the forefront of scientific and legislative debates.[35]

In particular, here, our problem relates to deficiencies in genetic ethics and public policy-making with reference to social ontology. Additionally, there are further problems even where such ethical principles and public policies do exist in some developed form, for they are often either found wanting or else they exist alongside and even compete with a series of conflicting and incompatible social ontologies. As Goodin *et al.* have argued, this problem further impacts upon issues such as consent, consultation and the identification of communities directly affected by genetic research: 'Bioethicists and

34 Cf. the now infamous 'Deaf Parent Hypothesis', a case study based upon a true story, where a couple trying for a baby had expressed the wish to give birth *only* to a deaf baby – because both parents were profoundly deaf. Hence they wished to abort any foetus which would have full or nearly full hearing. This case, along with the studies based upon it, often causes outrage. Yet for many who look beyond what I would call the 'societal imperative' that often dominates our thinking in such matters, this case is, in terms of ethics, no different from a situation where a couple who both have full hearing might wish to abort any foetus which showed signs of being deaf. In social, communitarian and ethical terms, there is no fundamental difference between the two.

35 Although space does not permit its detailed treatment here, we should also take note that another major area of concern is that of race. Issues here include debates surrounding the *social* construction of race, along with the biological influence upon (and justifications offered for) such construction, and the subsequent implications of this (in terms of issues such as genetic and other forms of discrimination, or issues of healthcare, equal opportunities and so on). On the social construction of race, see Joseph L. Graves, *The Emperor's New Clothes*, 2001; and S. S.-J. Lee, J. Mountain and B. A. Koenig, 'The Meanings of "Race" in the New Genomics: Implications for Health Disparities Research', *Yale Journal of Health Policy, Law and Ethics* 1, 2001, pp.33−75.

policymakers have argued over how best to define communities and have made varied recommendations for how researchers might consult the communities from which they hope to attract subjects.'[36]

Furthermore, this is not simply a problem posed by the development of pre-implantation genetic screening. It is obviously also an issue with regard to prenatal diagnosis (where there is a known risk to the foetus) and prenatal screening (where there is no known risk)[37] – the implications have simply been exacerbated by developments in PGD.

As Adrienne Asch, amongst others,[38] has argued, it is obvious that many researchers and policymakers do not consult such communities and, even where they do so, such consultation is frequently inadequate, too limited and often misinterpreted to the detriment of the community and its members alike. Elsewhere, Asch has highlighted figures which suggest that, in the last twenty years, a majority of the US parents whose health insurance covered the process have availed themselves of prenatal genetic screening. Those who have not done so on moral grounds constitute a very small minority and are perceived to be burdening society with a whole range of unnecessary problems. Such 'resisters' to the tide of the powerfully prevailing opinion come under increasing pressure from insurance companies, from doctors and even from members of their own families.[39] Indeed,

---

36   Holly C. Goodin, Benjamin Wilfond, Karina Boehm, and Barbara Bowles Biesecker, 'Unintended Messages: The Ethics of Teaching Genetic Dilemmas', *Hastings Center Report* 32, 2002, p.37.

37   For a definition of the two techniques and the difference between them, see Ford, *The Prenatal Person*, chapter 7, 'Prenatal Screening and Diagnosis', pp.121–43, especially pp.123–25. Significantly, Ford notes that 'most birth defects are not genetic', ibid., p.124.

38   See the work of those associated with 'The Disability Rights Critique of Prenatal Testing': http://lgruen.web.wesleyan.edu/wescourses/2003s/biol118/01/disabilityrights.pdf. Although Asch is usually primarily associated with the 'disability rights critique' of genetic medicine, her arguments have a much wider range of application in the debates that this present chapter deals with.

39   Adrienne Asch 'Prenatal testing: Implications for Family and Society', paper presented to the *Teaching the Ethical, Legal and Social Implications of the Human Genome* summer institute, Ethics Institute, Dartmouth College, USA, August 2003.

Asch indicates that many in the US now believe it likely that prenatal screening will become compulsory as part of a national healthcare policy (with increased selective abortion and '*in-vitro* action' – Asch's phrase – following as a result of the screening).[40]

In Asch's opinion (though note she describes herself as normally being 'pro-choice' in the abortion debate) these are worrying developments, because, whilst the seeking of prenatal testing may be based upon reasonable desires, the practice actually tends towards a lack of recognition of the uniqueness and unique value of *all* children (and hence, we might add, it logically follows that this impacts upon the unique value of all human beings).[41]

And here we come close to the heart of the matter. The subjective decision made (as the result of PGD or prenatal diagnosis or screening) to discard particular embryos or to abort certain foetuses in such cases is normally made against the backdrop of some imagined 'template' of what it is to be a 'normal' person, or to be as near as possible to some conception of a 'desirable citizen', or of a 'near-perfect' or even 'ideal' human person (whatever the denials that routinely surface in such debates). When it comes to certain diseases or disabilities, many today perceive (or even subconsciously come to view) the potential children who would 'suffer' from such 'limitation' as being 'lesser human beings' in value (and this sort of thinking bears striking parallels to that of the prominent eugenicists in the early to mid-twentieth century). But such thinking is heavily misguided. For we all have so-called flaws (that some might call 'imperfections') and, as Asch continues, we all, in some way, will have disappointed our parents – a disability is only one factor amongst so many to be taken into consideration here. Disabilities *can* be dealt with. All children have sets of characteristics which the family and society need to deal with. Disabilities are no different in this respect.[42] John Habgood has made a similar case from within a Christian context: 'Creation … endows another being with the freedom to be itself, with all the risks

40   Ibid.
41   Ibid.
42   Ibid.

and disappointments that might entail.'[43] Let us unpack the issues involved here a little further.

In an ongoing debate with Green, Asch has contended that, all too often, having a disability is deemed to be incompatible with life satisfaction. She believes that, all too frequently, many ethicists, researchers and those aligned with the health professions, along with the insurance industry and the public policy-making sectors, perceive a particular disability as *the* defining characteristic of any individual or group of individuals. She analyses contrasting 'medical and social paradigms of disability' and expresses similar concerns to those that I have already mentioned in the context of subjective interpretation and decision making in relation to 'quality of life'. Yet Asch wishes to highlight the fact that '... most of the problems associated with having a disability stem from discriminatory social arrangements that are changeable.'[44]

So, on the one hand, certainly some of those who work in (or are involved in the legislation on) medicine, genetic science and public health erroneously believe that people with disabilities might never enjoy a rewarding life and, on the other, they err in perceiving that any problems with which disabled people are confronted are 'attributable to the condition itself rather than to external factors'.[45] The alarming outcome of such beliefs and their influence upon policy-making and bioethics itself is that the emphasis tends towards ensuring that fewer people with such disabilities ever come into existence, as opposed to attempting to improve the lives of those who have or might develop certain disabilities:

---

43   John Habgood, 'Test-tube Idolatry', *The Tablet*, 2 August 2003, p.6. Obviously not all disabilities impact upon individuals and their families in an equal fashion, but this does not affect the main arguments under consideration here.

44   Adrienne Asch, 'Prenatal Diagnosis and Selective Abortion: A Challenge to Practice and Policy', *American Journal of Public Health* 89, November 1999, p.1650. None of this is to ignore that social provision for disabled people did improve considerably in many societies throughout the twentieth century. It is to point out that current developments could have a regressive effect upon such advances, as well as to indicate that efforts to improve the social lot of those with disabilities still have a very long way to go.

45   Ibid., p.1651.

> What differentiates prenatal testing followed by abortion from other forms of
> disability prevention and medical treatment is that prenatal testing followed by
> abortion is intended not to prevent the disability or illness of a born or future
> human being but *to prevent the birth of a human being who will have one of
> these undesired characteristics.*[46]

Asch also believes that the rationale for such prenatal diagnosis and selective abortion (and, presumably, discarding of embryos) is largely economic: the costs of childhood and later disability might somehow be lessened if each unborn child diagnosed as having a disability were to be aborted (or, we might go on to add, if 'defective' embryos were not implanted). In addition, some argue that the social, familial and societal 'costs' are also thereby reduced. Yet, with regard to all such 'costs', Asch constructs a convincing case to demonstrate that this is not only wishful thinking (or casuistry of an immoral kind) but is also factually very mistaken. Her analysis here merits being quoted at some length:

> On both empirical and moral grounds, endorsing prenatal diagnosis for societal
> reasons is dangerous. Only a small fraction of total disability can now be
> detected prenatally, and even if future technology enables the detection of
> predisposition to diabetes, forms of depression, Alzheimer diseases, heart
> disease, arthritis, or back problems – all more prevalent than many of the
> currently detectable conditions – we will never manage to detect and prevent
> most disability. Rates of disability increase markedly with age, and the gains in
> life span guarantee that most people will deal with disability in themselves or
> someone close to them. Laws and services to support people with disabilities
> will still be necessary, unless society chooses a campaign of eliminating
> disabled people in addition to preventing the births of those who would be
> disabled. Thus, there is small cost-saving in money or in human resources to be
> achieved by even the vigorous determination to test every pregnant woman and
> abort every fetus found to exhibit disabling traits.[47]

Here we identify a further key issue in our deliberations, for we are thus able to identify a tendency for certain interest groups, organisations, theorists, researchers and ethicists to say, in effect, that it is

46   Ibid., p.1651 (my italics).
47   Ibid., p.1652.

better for certain individuals (and therefore for the community which they together could constitute) *not to be.*

And yet, even on such crude economic grounds, or even on genuinely empathetic or compassionate grounds, such reasoning is highly flawed. We cannot overlook that many arguments in such cases are shaped by economic, expedient or immoral (or at best amoral) motivating factors. Further, it has been shown that any supposed benefits to society in general from such policies are questionable.[48] But, beyond any such motivating factors, this reasoning would appear to be based largely upon the highly subjective and much contested 'quality of life' criteria mentioned earlier.

Asch believes that society should instead acknowledge that disabled people bring many riches to the lives of others, and she asserts that, above all else, a life with a disability is a worthwhile life. Indeed, disability 'precludes far fewer life possibilities than [some] members of the bioethics community claim'.[49] As stated, most of the problems impeding the lives of disabled persons actually have social, rather than biological, causes. Indeed, as Asch illustrates, many of those who would advocate the widespread screening of foetuses and the abortion of those diagnosed with disabilities tend to ignore the evidence, coming from families with disabled persons within them, of how enhancing and enriching the childhood and later lives of those disabled individuals can be. Many of those involved with medicine, bioethics, healthcare and insurance, as well as public policy making, have proved to be ignorant and misinformed with regard to the true nature of life with a disability.

Thus Asch wishes to propose that society should adapt to fit those who exist, rather than declaring that 'some people should not exist because society is not prepared for them'.[50] If society is ready to accept children with disabilities and is welcoming to them or, as Asch puts it, if the child is 'not a problem for the world, and the world is not

---

48   Indeed, just as the supposed financial benefits of stem cell technologies have, according to recent studies, been grossly exaggerated; see reports in *The Economist*, 22 September 2005.

49   Asch, 'Prenatal Diagnosis and Selective Abortion', p.1652.

50   Ibid., p.1655.

a problem for the child',[51] then there will be no need for such wide-spread prenatal screening and the resulting abortions. None of this is to underestimate or simplify the enormity of the challenges that are faced by families caring for severely handicapped children.

This debate between Green and Asch helps us to identify and draw together a number of important issues for those concerned with the interrelation between the ethics of community and the ethics of genetics. Not least among these is the question of whether aspects of genetic science and medicine and their resulting social effects are actually eugenics under another name, as Asch and others appear to imply.

A second major issue is that of the discrimination against certain individuals and communities which is emerging as a result of such scientific, medical and even bioethical developments. In the first study of its kind, an Australian federal government-funded *Genetic Discrimination Project* survey of 1185 people who had willingly subjected themselves to genetic testing[52] found that 438 reported that their having undergone testing had led to their being disadvantaged, with 87 reporting discrimination at the hands of doctors, insurance companies, employers and even close relatives or spouses. However, the problem here is that the very concept of 'genetic discrimination' is still one which has not received full attention in all quarters concerned either with the genetic research itself or with the policies which follow from legal and political deliberations upon its implications.[53]

The social and communitarian issues raised by examples such as these, along with the transformation in social values and norms, illustrate that there is a need for these relationships between the ethics

---

51 Ibid., p.1656. See also Adrienne Asch, 'Why I Haven't Changed My Mind about Prenatal Diagnosis: Reflections and Refinements', in *Prenatal Testing and Disability Rights*, ed. Erik Parens and Adrienne Asch (Washington DC: Georgetown University Press, 2000), pp.234–58, where Asch develops and refines her arguments further.

52 The tests in question here ranged from those for certain forms of breast cancer, to Huntington's disease, to haemochromatosis. The work of the project moved beyond the initial investigative stages in January 2006. Its ongoing work can be followed through its reports at: www.gdproject.org.

53 See Lisa N. Geller, 'Current Developments in Genetic Discrimination'.

of community and the ethics of genetics to be explored in much more detail. Hence there is need for far greater ethical consideration in all debates concerning developments in genetics and, in turn, for less primacy to be accorded to economic and scientific factors.

Conclusions

I hope that the material we have considered demonstrates that dispari-ties between the ethics of genetics and the ethics of community are a cause for concern. Let me close by considering possible further areas of specific concern, the investigation and exploration of which might yet further inform the ethics of genetics in relation to community.

Perhaps what has been implicit throughout this chapter might now become more explicit: it is worth reiterating that I believe that very specific and valuable contributions can be offered to all these debates and dilemmas by the moral sub-disciplines within theology and philosophy that relate to *pedagogical* issues in this field; as well as to the debates surrounding perceived differences in method, *telos* and delivery between 'applied' and 'professional' ethics. In particular, practitioners in these disciplines might seek to counter the 'scientific fundamentalism' which breeds an intolerance of ethical, religious and communitarian perspectives that appear to place restrictions upon aspects of research and technological development.[54]

This volume as a whole, it is hoped, illustrates that truly fruitful dialogue between different disciplines is not only possible but can

54   One welcome example in relation to the issue of social ontology is Frank G. Kirkpatrick, *A Moral Ontology for a Theistic Ethic: Gathering the Nations in Love and Justice* (Harmondsworth, Ashgate, 2003). Here, see also the work of the Genetics, Theology and Ethics Group being convened by Lisa Sowle Cahill and J. Donald Monan of Boston College, USA (published by Continuum in 2005) and the ongoing and considerable contributions made by Celia Deane-Drummond, herself trained as a scientist, who has made numerous and highly significant contributions across a wide range of ethical discussions pertaining to science, medicine and the environment.

take a wide variety of forms and have some pleasantly surprising results, as all involved find themselves to be enriched and that their own perspectives are widened and enhanced.

Questions concerning the ethics of genetics

Given our foregoing considerations, it appears that there may be a 'chicken and egg' dilemma at work in genetic research and medicine today; and so, also, in the public policies which they influence. On the one hand, research is often conducted by persons without adequate training or interest in the ethical issues involved, and on the other, there are difficulties involved with ethicists having to foresee potential moral dilemmas that might only occur in the future.

So there is a need to ask how many decisions involving genetics and the effects of the Human Genome project are based upon highly subjective grounds (whether influenced by personal factors, political bodies and processes, the media or particular interest groups) in the guise of objective grounds (when the default should be to attempt to approximate to as objective a decision as possible, in all scenarios). In particular, what decisions are based upon a subjective concept of the 'quality of life'? Of course, some would object that there is no alternative to subjective grounds, and argue that the 'sanctity of life' is no less subjective than the 'quality of life'. Even if this could be proved to be the case, the 'sanctity of life' grounding for ethical deliberation errs on the side of caution, is more universalistic in the application and nature of the justice it seeks to encourage, and is more amenable to the harmony and flourishing of communities. Indeed, it has stood the test of time and diverse application rather better than has the 'quality of life' principle.[55]

Quality of life *is* important and highly relevant to ethical debates, but taken in isolation as a guide for decision- and policy-making it can

---

55   Furthermore, recent debates in natural law theory (particularly the proportionalism debate) and in virtue ethics, suggest that it can still prove much more effective than the often crudely utilitarian nature of the 'quality of life' principle (taken in isolation).

be detrimental to individuals and societies alike. As John Elford, Ann Marie Mealey and Adam Hood illustrate in different ways elsewhere in this volume, there are much broader considerations to bear in mind when trying to reach important decisions about scientific, medical and legislative policy and practice. Stephen Bellamy offers an incisive case study to further illustrate this fundamentally important point. Gareth Jones contributes widely to the cumulative arguments that the book as a whole makes for having more than the simple expediency of 'quality of life' as the basis for our contemporary ethics.

To their voices I shall add but a plea that ethics might form an ever-increasing component of all courses in science, medicine and law; and that regular refresher training in ethics (and in applied ethics in particular) should become mandatory for all those engaged in these professions. Many strides have been taken towards such developments in recent years, but perhaps it is time for more legislation and for funding to be made available, so that ethical training might become the norm across the board.

Furthermore, in regard to the 'quality of life' debates, the rights of certain individuals and communities and the increasing prevalence of genetic discrimination, we must also ask who decides, shapes and influences what is perceived to be a 'normal' human being? Numerous problems arise from the fact that many engaged with the ethics of genetics are working with differing and even competing methods of ethics, and that individuals have recourse to several schools of moral thought that are not always compatible. Indeed, much of the evidence under consideration would point towards a judgement that, in many cases, human persons, foetuses and embryos are being viewed as simply 'means to ends' as opposed to being 'ends in themselves'.

Social, familial and communitarian questions

Here we return to the world of *Gattaca* which, in itself, was really an image of the eugenicists' ideal society projected onto the future. It should not, however, be allowed to become *our* future. Whether we like it or not, or wish to confront it or not, there is a real danger that certain advances in genetic technology could lead to the creation of a new genetic 'underclass' or to a number of new classes, groups or communities being excluded from the benefits enjoyed by mainstream society. There are potentially drastic consequences of genetic technology upon families in particular, which have still further implications for wider communities and societies in general.

Certain groups are or may become increasingly stigmatised or re-stigmatised as a result of developments in genetics. For example, sufferers from achondroplasia in the case of the latter or sufferers from heart disease or alcoholism in the former. There is a real possibility that we will see a major increase in the number and range of services, healthcare benefits and insurance cover that are denied to certain individuals and groups of individuals or communities. Again, those deemed to have 'undesirable' characteristics when compared with any prevailing template of the 'desirable' citizen will suffer accordingly.

Untrammelled and unchecked, unregulated or merely quasi-regulated (in the fashion that we have come to despair about as the norm in contemporary Britain and like societies), such technological and scientific developments pose a genuine risk of the further fragmentation of community life as so many know and value it (or at least aspire towards it). Will advances in genetic technology lead to the ever greater prevalence of individualistic thinking and the gradual demise of ontological thinking, beyond its reference to the individual alone?

There are serious failings in many of the dominant social ontologies currently prevailing. Indeed, our considerations lead me to suggest that it appears there is a general vacuum in genetic ethics with regards to the very field of social ontology itself. Yet only a clearly defined conception of community-oriented social ontology, and a firm defence of this conception, can counter the ethically negative implications of such an overt focus upon the individual.

Unless all such discussions and investigations are carried out as thoroughly as possible, and all voices listened to, the negative and discriminatory tendencies of the eugenics of old could easily rise again and have a major impact upon certain communities and their individual members, leading to a further breakdown in social cohesion (even in a surreptitious fashion and, so to speak, by the 'back door').

It is beyond doubt that the technology we have been speaking about can be exploited for unethical purposes.

Hence we need to give greater attention to all the ways in which social norms, values and judgements can be significantly transformed as a result of the genetic revolution. We need to discern whether each such transformation is, in the main, positive or negative from a communitarian perspective.

Otherwise, things that we value so highly, such as learning, love and socialisation, as well as familial and communitarian obligations and co-operation, will become less important – they might all be 'short circuited' in consequence of genetic technology. Children are in danger of becoming more like commodities (even status symbols) in the wake of both actual and potential advances in genetic technology. As Hilary and Steven Rose argue (drawing attention to fears also expressed by John Habgood):

> We are witnessing a process that increasingly turns a child into a commodity, with product specification, quality control and rejection of sub-standard products – the wrong sex, the wrong genes. The process also harms the clinicians who, instead of being professionals who give the best advice regardless of market considerations, become the providers of biotechnical services to customers with effective demand powers.[56]

So we should strive to consider our reaction to such developments, long before the scientific and legislative agendas have left ethics behind. So, too, the impact of scientific developments upon communities should always be borne in mind at the earliest possible stage of debate. Hence, this is my plea to place the ethical horse before the legislative cart and, in turn, the legislative horse before the scientific cart. Some might argue that this would hinder science or involve ethicists gazing into crystal balls to predict the future implications of scientific advances. Not at all – ethics has always been concerned

---

56   Hilary and Steven Rose, 'Playing God', *The Guardian*, 3 July 2003, p.25. They take Baroness Warnock to task for her flippant acceptance of proposals to take eggs from aborted foetuses, as she could not see any problems for the mother. The Roses comment that: 'It is distressing to find a social philosopher who has contributed so much to this debate forgetting the children', ibid.

with assessing hypothetical as well as real-life scenarios and, as we see with films such as *Gattaca*, many in society are very adept at perceiving the potential pitfalls of the permissive and minimal ethical regulation of science and medicine.

Part Three: Regulation and Policy

D. GARETH JONES

Regulatory Procedures

Introduction

The biomedical procedures considered in this book have a dominant characteristic, and this is their applied nature. They have social ramifications, they will be applied in real life situations, and the manner in which they are applied is open to adaptation and extension. One of the procedures considered here, namely PGD, was originally introduced with serious single gene disorders in mind. However, its use has been extended in a number of directions, including the detection of late onset genetic conditions. Regardless of the ethical issues raised by such applications, they typify a common phenomenon – the initial applications will never remain the only ones. More radical applications will almost inevitably arise, sometimes far removed from the original ones and generally driven by social pressures. For their part, these pressures usually have a much weaker therapeutic rationale than did the original applications.

These observations are pertinent to the subject of this chapter, since regulatory procedures have to contend with this ever-changing social landscape. They also have to accommodate the diversity of ethical and social viewpoints encountered within pluralist societies. It is into this seething milieu that most of us arrive with our well, or inadequately, formulated theological and ethical stances. How do we cope, and what contribution, if any, can we make to the ongoing and exceedingly vigorous debate?

In an attempt to throw some light on this debate, two contrasting examples will be examined here, both of them from the reproductive area. The first revolves around what we can and cannot do to and with human embryos. The second centres on IVF surrogacy. In each case, what options do societies have?

Embryo Research and Embryonic Stem Cells

Research on human embryos can take a number of forms, with a number of goals. The derivation of embryonic stem cells (ESCs) from embryos is one of these, although in future it could have a therapeutic rationale rather than a purely research one. Whilst research *per se* on human embryos is not identical with ESC procedures, they have much in common and so can be taken together, since currently the process of obtaining ESCs from embryos destroys those embryos. In other words, research on human embryos and deriving ESCs both lead to embryonic death. What significance do societies attach to this, and how protective are they of human embryos in the laboratory?

Debate on these questions normally revolves around the moral status of the human embryo. However, it should be evident by now that there is no way in which pluralist societies will reach any consensus on this issue. The usual positions will be rehearsed: complete protection of the embryo, no protection of any description, and a raft of intermediate positions seeking some protection. In practice, it is the latter stance, with its attempt to strike a balance between competing goods, that emerges as the crucial one in regulations.

Societies, of course, also have regulations governing human life under other circumstances. These include *in vitro* fertilisation (IVF) and the associated production of large numbers of surplus embryos, contraceptive devices and drugs (some of which act by preventing implantation of embryos), and abortion. These other regulations raise the question of the requirement for consistency between policies governing human life in its early stages. Is it ethically acceptable to allow embryo destruction under one set of circumstances but ban it under another set? Is consistency of stance not an ethical, and perhaps a theological, requirement?

While a large number of positions and sub-positions regarding society's valuation and utilisation of embryos can be discerned, four dominant ones emerge, which have been categorised as A, B, C and D in these terms:[1]

A. banning the use of embryos in research, and banning the use of established human ESCs in research;
B. banning the use of embryos in research, but allowing the use of established human ESCs in at least some research;
C. allowing the use of surplus IVF embryos in research, and allowing the derivation of human ESCs and their subsequent use in research;
D. allowing the use not only of surplus IVF embryos in research but also of embryos created specifically for research purposes, and allowing the derivation of human ESCs from either, and also their subsequent use in research.

Position A

This stance is based on the argument that the human embryo is a moral person from fertilisation onwards, and so can be benefited or harmed, just like us. Consequently, embryo research does nothing less than destroy human lives. Thus, position A prohibits all human embryo research, including the extraction and use of ESCs.

Ireland, Austria, Norway and Poland take this position. Ireland has no specific legislation regarding embryo research or the use of human ESCs. However, its constitution implicitly prohibits research on the embryo, as the State 'acknowledges the right to life of the unborn' and 'guarantees in its laws to respect, and, as far as practicable, by its laws to defend and vindicate that right'.[2]

A recent report on IVF practices in Ireland almost unanimously recommended that surplus embryos created via IVF be permitted to be used for research and that embryos created *in vitro* be given legal pro-

---

1   C. R. Towns and D. G. Jones, 'Stem cells: public policy and ethics', *New Zealand Bioethics Journal* 5, 2004, pp.22–28.
2   Constitution of Ireland (Bunreacht na hÉireann), Article 40, par.3.

tection only when placed in a woman's body.[3] However, experiment-ation on embryos, or their destruction, is generally considered to be unacceptable, and it appears unlikely that embryo or ESC research will be permitted in Ireland in the near future.

Position B

Countries whose policy falls into position B confine the use of ESCs to those currently in existence. What this means is that the ESC lines are already established, the ESCs having been extracted prior to a specified date, (the date being determined by when the legislation is approved by parliament). This ensures that no ESCs can be extracted at any future date. This is what might be termed a 'modified pro-hibition' stance. ESC research can be pursued, but within stringent limits, namely, utilising only existing cell lines. This position is an attempt to achieve a balance between protecting the human embryo and preventing its commodification, and allowing some research using ESCs.

Germany is an example of a country that takes this position. Any use of an embryo 'not suiting its own preservation' is banned in Germany under the Embryo Protection Act 1990. However, this does not include ESCs, which are covered by the Stem Cell Act 2002. This latter bans, as a matter of principle, the importation and utilisation of ESCs. However, exceptions to the ban are allowed if the ESCs were derived before 1 January 2002 from surplus IVF embryos. These can be imported, as long as they were obtained in accordance with the relevant national legislation in the country of origin and if no compensation has been made for the donation of the embryos. ESC research may only be carried out where the research is considered worthwhile and if it cannot be carried out using animals or any other type of cell.

3   Department of Health and Children, *Report of the Commission on Assisted Human Reproduction.* Available from: http://www.dohc.ie/publications/cahr. html, 2005.

Position C

This position allows for the use and ongoing isolation of ESCs from embryos surplus to the requirements of clinical IVF programmes. This is a 'modified acceptance' stance. While there is no attempt to bestow absolute protection upon the embryo, there are restrictions as to the origin of all embryos used in any process. Surplus IVF embryos are those that have been created for potential implantation into a woman but are no longer required for reproductive purposes. Consequently, most of these will ultimately be destroyed, though an extremely small number are donated to other couples for reproductive purposes. Ethically, the ideal is to separate completely the decision to destroy surplus embryos from the decision to use them for research.[4] The rationale for this stipulation is to demonstrate a degree of respect for the human embryo, while encouraging research that may benefit future patients.

Although legislation on these matters in Australia has undergone changes over the last few years, and intense debate is continuing, it currently serves as an example of a country that takes this position.[5] Research may be carried out on any ESC line derived from surplus IVF embryos. Therapeutic cloning is banned, as is reproductive cloning. This position was challenged by the 2005 Lockhart review, which proposed a series of liberalising recommendations, including permitting therapeutic cloning and the creation of animal-human hybrids.[6] However, the Australian parliament is unlikely to go along with these recommendations.

---

4   D. G. Jones and C. R. Towns, 'Navigating the quagmire: the regulation of human embryonic stem cell research', *Human Reproduction* 21, 2006, pp. 1113–16.

5   Research Involving Human Embryos Act 2002; Prohibition of Human Cloning Act 2002.

6   Legislation Review Committee, 'Reports on the Prohibition of Human Cloning Act 2002 and the Research Involving Human Embryos Act 2002', 19 December 2005. Available at: http://www.lockhartreview.com.au/public/content/ViewCategory.aspx?id=35.

Position D

Countries adopting position D permit the creation of human embryos specifically for research purposes, either via somatic cell nuclear transfer (SCNT, cloning) or by IVF fertilisation. This is in addition to allowing the use of surplus IVF embryos. In other words, this position represents a 'broader acceptance' stance. Note however that, apart from this additional source of embryos, positions C and D are identical. Nevertheless, this move from the use of already existing embryos to ones brought into existence specifically for research purposes is seen by many as crossing a fundamental ethical dividing-line.

The United Kingdom is a position D country, where embryos can be created for research purposes as long as the proposed research falls within a number of clearly defined categories. These include basic biological research, fertility research, research directed towards the prevention of hereditary diseases or towards the curing of serious adult diseases. This means that ESCs can be derived from embryos in each of these instances so long as they are accepted as being crucial to the research. All research is licensed and monitored by the Human Fertilisation and Embryology Authority (HFEA). The first licence to create embryos for research was issued in August 2004, although to date most of the embryo research that has been carried out has used surplus IVF embryos.

Theological Aspects

These policy issues are matters to which theologians have given little attention in years past. To an extent this is quite understandable. After all, any theological implications of stem cells would not have been foreseeable prior to their therapeutic and research potential becoming a subject of interest to scientists. Hence, this is territory that is as startlingly new for theologians as it is for everyone else. Are there existing theological principles and models that might help us resolve these exceedingly complex dilemmas?

An obvious place to seek such assistance would be within the context provided by the abortion debate. After all, the crux of this debate is the moral status of the foetus, with its clear parallel with the moral status of the embryo. However, there are two limitations. The first is that the relationship between the foetus within a mother's uterus and the much less developed early embryo in the laboratory is far from direct. This is the contrast between an 8–20 week gestation foetus and a less than 14 day embryo (frequently a 5–7 day blastocyst). There is no reason why a standpoint on abortion should be directly translated into the same standpoint on embryo research. The second limitation is that the many other considerations relevant to abortion in the one instance and embryo research in the other also have to be taken into account. These considerations are quite different in the two cases. Unfortunately, therefore, theological reflection has little in the way of historical precedents to which it can look.

At a more general level, dominating motifs have tended to be those of playing God and designing children, motifs that have been interpreted negatively by many (but not all) theologians. While details of these do not concern us here, their negative connotations have led many theological commentators to adopt a biased stance against embryo research and the use of ESCs. This has had profound repercussions for the policy debates we are considering, with theologians tending towards positions A or B and away from C and D.

In this environment it is easy to lose sight of other aspects of a Christian perspective, namely, its emphasis upon the intentions and motives of researchers, clinicians and patients. How are these to be incorporated into each of these positions? Might they lead to an open-endedness not usually found in bioethical and policy discussions? Where, too, do we fit in the possibility that research might elevate our concept of humans as beings made in the image of God?

Whatever view we emerge with on the respective merits of the four positions, we should also look closely at our character as people before God. Specific answers will depend on a close analysis of ethical and scientific considerations, but only within the context of how we act as people seeking to live as God's worthy stewards. We need to ask repeatedly what might be in the best interests of those for whom we have responsibility.

Keeping these general background considerations in mind, we should now ask whether any of the four positions have any theological correlates. What contribution can theology make to the formulation of policy here?[7]

Position A is compatible with the stance that human life commences at fertilisation, allowing nothing to be done to the embryo that is not in its own best interests. Such a stance would be expected also to disapprove of IVF, as both its development and practice necessitate the destruction of embryos. This position will not facilitate any research or subsequent therapy dependent upon the use of ESCs. Consequently, its emphasis is entirely on the harm done to embryos, ignoring the good that might accrue to others in the human community through the therapeutic potential of ESCs. From a Christian perspective this appears to fail to do justice to the obligations of servanthood, living in community, loving our neighbours as ourselves, and seeking to bring healing and wholeness to those in need. Focusing exclusively on one segment of the community (embryos) might entail acting unjustly towards other segments. Admittedly, there are many Christian commentators who will disagree with this assessment, although it may be noted that an exclusively pro-embryo stance does have side-effects frequently ignored in the theological literature.

It is against this background that position B appears particularly attractive. By allowing potentially beneficial research only on ESC lines already in existence, position B permits some research on human embryos while simultaneously aiming to protect human embryos. Since the embryos in question have already been destroyed, utilisation of extant stem cells in scientific research has much to commend it in communitarian terms. This position requires one to walk a moral tightrope: accepting the destruction of some embryos, while arguing against the destruction of others; preventing some research but accepting other research.

How should this compromise position be viewed theologically? Christians who view moral personhood as originating at fertilisation

---

7   D. G. Jones, 'Why should cloning and stem cell research be of interest to theologians?', in *Stem Cell Research and Cloning*, ed. D. Gareth Jones and Mary Byrne (Adelaide: ATF Press, 2004), pp.73–94.

have reacted in two contrasting ways. For some, the position is too liberal, since it accepts embryo destruction as legitimate, even though the destruction occurred in the past. For them, position A is thus the only theologically acceptable position. A second perspective has welcomed the compromise position as a way of taking science seriously while also protecting the interests of embryos. In other words, there is difference of opinion even within the more conservative schools of theological thought. Whether or not the difference is theologically rooted is another matter.

However, there is a problem with consistency of policy in those societies that permit IVF programmes that produce surplus embryos. The restrictive ESC guidelines of position B fail to protect the large numbers of surplus IVF embryos that are routinely destroyed within IVF programmes. For those who value the personhood of embryos from fertilisation onwards, position A is the more consistent of the two positions. Nevertheless, it does have repercussions in other areas of policy; repercussions that have to be weighed up theologically.

Position C provides limited protection of the human embryo, but this is within the framework of a more consistent ethical stance. Embryo research is limited to surplus IVF embryos, with a procedural separation between the initial decision to discard embryos and the subsequent decision to donate them for research. This allows both the utilisation and extraction of new ESCs, and eliminates arbitrary time limits on extraction.

Aside from its consistency, position C also fulfils a broad range of Christian imperatives, seeking to improve the health status of numerous individuals suffering from common debilitating conditions, as well treating early embryos with the care and respect due to human tissue. It is true that it opens the door to the destruction of early embryos, but this is done within a framework of previously agreed destruction. The research is on embryos that have no future as human individuals. This emphasis is theologically commendable, being on that which is best for the human community. As such it deserves serious consideration by Christians.

But what about the creation of embryos for research purposes, either by IVF or SCNT, and the move to position D? This represents a shift in moral perspective, since embryos are being created specifically for research purposes; there is no intention that they will ever develop into human individuals. Here the destruction of embryos is premeditated and there can be no separation of the decision to destroy the embryo and the decision to use it for research. This is generally seen as a massive shift in moral, let alone theological, perspective. Whether or not this is the case is becoming the focus of increasingly interesting debate, since there may be inconsistency in allowing the production of surplus embryos in IVF but rejecting the research possibilities represented by position D. The result in both instances is the creation and destruction of embryos. Nevertheless, this is a position that at present finds very little favour among theological commentators.

Challenges for Communities, including Theological Communities

In one country after another, debates over legislative regulations are ongoing and constantly changing. These changes mirror the increasing understanding of the nature of the scientific developments and their clinical potential. Additionally, as initial reluctance to embrace the procedures is replaced by gradual acceptance, the tenor of the debates shifts. This movement may manifest itself as what may be interpreted as a liberalising drift from one position to another. Once position B is accepted, position C appears more tolerable; and once position C is taken, embracing position D becomes conceivable.

For some, this shift is a perfect illustration of the slippery slope, as the prohibitive regime of position A gives way to less and less prohibitive stances, ending up with the creation of embryos solely for research purposes and position D. However, distinct issues and distinct responses characterise each position, and each has to be argued on its own merits. The move beyond position A does *not* inevitably lead to position D. In other words, it is conceivable that this 'drift' is, in fact, a principled shift.

Regardless of the nature of the regulations under the microscope, they are subject to a host of liberalising pressures within societies. While these pressures are frequently scientific or technological in origin ('if something can be done it should be done'), they may be social pressures ('it is my right to have access to this new procedure'). There is no escape from pressures like these in the debates over embryo research and the use of ESCs. Although these debates are invariably conducted against a backdrop of positions on the moral status of the embryo, this is merely one ingredient, as evidenced by what I have termed the principled drift in a liberalising direction. The other ingredients are fuelled by scientific and therapeutic considerations, the new vistas opened up by increased understanding of early embryonic development, and growing awareness of the stances taken by societies on the relative value of human embryos in other reproductive contexts. While these pressures may, in part, originate from scientists, they also emanate from ordinary citizens who (rightly or wrongly) perceive benefits for themselves and their families in the exploitation of ESCs.

Scientists are not alone in wanting to forge ahead into new realms; they are accompanied far more than is often appreciated by the communities of which they (and we) are a part. As human beings, we seek to better our world, both personal and communal, and we turn increasingly to science to supply the solutions. Our expectations of what science can do for us have vastly expanded, as one advance after another has been made. Unfortunately, these expectations are sometimes too high, since any clinical applications might be far more distant than anticipated. Yet even when science is able to achieve what we hope for, we still need to pause and question if it actually should go ahead. This is where the community's expectations come into play, expectations that may be open to social manipulation in any direction. Public opinion presents considerable challenges to those who formulate public policy, since its basis may be ephemeral. Should regulation be shaped by the desires of the public, or at least those who are vociferous in making their desires known, or should regulation dictate to society what policy makers consider acceptable?

Further, who makes the regulations and on what basis are they formulated? In particular, what contribution might theological think-

ing make? Inevitably, it is one voice among many, but is it a distinctive voice? As we have seen, there is a diversity of theological opinion
over embryo research and ESCs, most supporting positions A, B or C,
with far fewer advocating position D. This suggests that the theological voice is not a distinctive one – and perhaps it should not be
expected to be. Theologians contribute to the regulations that emerge,
rather than determine what they will be.

    In order to illustrate the complexities faced by societies, let alone
by Christian groups, in contributing to ethical regulation, let us consider IVF surrogacy.

A Regulatory Nightmare: IVF Surrogacy

It is worthwhile pondering IVF surrogacy because at one level it is not
technically demanding, neither is it particularly sophisticated, and so
one might imagine that the ethical issues would be straightforward.
And yet this is far from the case, since what we have here is a clear
illustration of the way in which society's expectations are changing
very rapidly. And it is these changes that are proving ethically problematic, rather than any unexpected technological developments that
appear to pose new challenges to our view of the moral status of, let
us say, the embryo.

    Over recent years in New Zealand, a national ethics committee
has borne the brunt of these developments, as it has the responsibility
of assessing, on a case-by-case basis, all surrogacy proposals that
involve a fertility clinic. The guidelines used to review IVF surrogacy
proposals contain a number of requirements that have to be met for
the application to be approved. These requirements are expressions of
the underlying ethical principles adopted by the committee.

    The first requirement is that surrogacy is restricted to 'non-com-
mercial surrogacy', on the premise that the intrusion of commercial
factors militates against any altruistic base. The motivations are expected to be altruistic in nature. From this it follows that the birth
mother may not be paid to enter into the surrogacy arrangement or

reimbursed for lost income during pregnancy. The fear here is that any such payment could be seen as making surrogacy a form of employment. However, the intending parents may cover expenses directly related to the pregnancy, such as travel or maternity wear. The fear that the child-to-be might be viewed as a commodity undoubtedly underlies this requirement, fuelled as this concern frequently is by scenarios of child-buying and child-selling, as too does the perception that human beings are being converted into items to be bought and sold on an open market.

At least one of the intending parents must be genetically related to the child-to-be; in other words, both donated sperm and donated ova cannot be used together. There also has to be a clearly defined medical reason preventing the intending mother from undertaking a pregnancy; alternatively, there has to be a medical diagnosis of infertility. This requirement is intended to exclude IVF surrogacy for purely social or convenience reasons.

Another set of requirements concerns the birth mother. She needs to be healthy, with no condition that would preclude a safe pregnancy and birth. The birth mother must also have completed her own family – the goal in this instance being to reduce the likelihood that she may want to keep the child she has carried. She should either be a family member or a close friend of the intending parents, with the added proviso that the friendship has preceded the surrogacy proposal. This has been considered imperative for a number of reasons. It helps to highlight the motive for surrogacy, that is, compassion as opposed to financial gain. Closely related to this is the goal of establishing a set of meaningful relationships for the child-to-be, including possibly with the birth mother, following the birth. The intention is also to assist the birth mother to cope with the loss of the child she has carried. Alongside these considerations is the intention of setting the stage for forming a robust agreement between the intending parents and the birth mother in the inevitable absence of any rigid or legally enforceable contract. In much the same vein, both the birth mother and the intending parents have to be permanent residents in New Zealand.

Further, the surrogacy application must include a report from legal advisers to ensure that the participants understand the associated legal issues. The application must also include reports from counsellors who have met with both family groups, including existing children. This is important in order to ascertain the specific issues associated with each situation, as well as any complications likely to arise and whether these have been addressed.

These guidelines were developed for a particular set of circumstances, and initially appeared robust. However, some applications have pushed the boundaries of what is considered a reasonable use of surrogacy, and the guidelines began to prove inadequate within one to two years of their formulation. Consider the following two cases.

In the first example, the intending parents already have three children but have always hoped to have more. However, this has been thwarted by the wife's need for an emergency hysterectomy following a Caesarean section for placenta previa at the time of her last delivery. The birth mother is the niece-in-law of the intending parents and there appears to be no coercion involved.

In many ways, this is relatively uncomplicated, although the intending parents already have three children of their own; they have not experienced infertility. The problem from their perspective is that they have been denied having a large family. This lies outside the current guidelines, since the meaning of infertility has been changed. What are the ethical implications of this, and to what extent should surrogacy and related technological procedures be used to satisfy a longing for a large family as opposed to a family?

In a second example, a couple find themselves unable to conceive either naturally or via multiple IVF attempts. They are desperate to conceive, and as they have been turned down for adoption they view surrogacy as their final option. Unable to find a surrogate from their own families, the intending parents place an advertisement in a newspaper, offering to cover all expenses. The potential birth parents respond to the advertisement in the newspaper, since the birth mother had previously been contemplating surrogacy, though had not discussed this desire with anyone. The intending parents and birth mother have now met face-to-face on three occasions, and claim to be in regular contact, saying that a friendship is forming. The birth mother and her partner feel compassion for the intending parents' situation. They live 400km from the intending parents.

This example begins to challenge the ethical guidelines under which IVF surrogacy proposals are currently assessed. There has been no ongoing relationship between the two parties prior to the appearance of the advertisement. In other words, the relationship between the intending parents and birth parents has sprung up solely within the context of surrogacy. It is highly questionable that there will be a meaningful ongoing relationship between the intending parents and birth mother following the birth of the child. While no commercial transaction has been hinted at, the use of an advertisement to initiate the surrogacy discussions has overtones of commodification.

These examples will suffice for giving some indication of the manner in which the original intentions behind IVF surrogacy are being stretched. Further complications have arisen when:

- intending parents advertise for a birth mother on the internet;
- intending parents and birth mother have never met;
- the birth mother lives in another country;
- intending parents are (male) homosexuals.

It is clear from these examples that the regulatory body is beset by liberalising pressures coming not from scientists or clinicians but from the applicants. These social pressures challenge the regulations by seeking to allow applications that increasingly diverge from the ones originally intended in the guidelines.

But were the original guidelines exemplary? Was their basis just? For instance, the financial assistance that the intending parents are permitted to provide to the birth mother may be unrealistically limited. Similarly, the stipulation requiring a pre-existing friendship between the intending parents and the birth mother has as its goal preservation of the priority of altruism, but the birth mother could have an altruistic motive in the absence of such a friendship. The guidelines assume that we naturally feel greater altruism towards the people whom we know and love than we do towards complete strangers; a generally safe assumption. However, it appears that there are women who genuinely desire to be surrogates for women they have not met. The altruism in such cases appears to arise out of empathy for the situation of the infertile couple, rather than out of a personal relationship. Should this be restricted?

This question is intensified when the possibility of repeat surrogacy arrangements is considered – could it then become a form of employment? There are reports of a woman in the United Kingdom who has been a surrogate eight times and is planning her ninth. This woman appears to enjoy being pregnant and helping infertile couples. The recompense she usually receives is significantly lower than the usual rate in UK surrogacy arrangements.[8]

Quite apart from the limitations of the most well-intentioned guidelines, the possibilities contemplated at one point in time may be rapidly overtaken by further possibilities previously never considered. These possibilities are generally of two types: scientific and social. An enormous amount of ethical debate surrounding artificial reproductive technologies concentrates on the manner in which scientific expectations become transformed with the passage of time, sometimes with major ethical consequences. The examples quoted here have nothing to do with scientific developments; they are all entirely social. The guidelines were developed within a particular social context, only to be overtaken within a very short period of time by radically different social expectations. Opening the door to one set of possibilities almost immediately opened it to further possibilities.

What this brings to light is the intimate interplay between ethics, science and society. What we have here is a very clear example of the way in which the uses to which a procedure are put may well change in response to social pressures, while the availability of the procedure itself may lead to yet further changes. This forces one to ask what role ethical guidelines actually play within this set of dynamic and interacting forces. It also shows why we have to take seriously the contention sometimes aired that bioethicists have failed to stop the inroads of liberalising tendencies into medicine in all its guises.

8   BBC News, 'New surrogate baby makes eight', 31 October 2002. Available at: http://news.bbc.co.uk/2/hi/uk_news/england/2382957.stm. Accessed on 21 May 2006.

What then can we say about the response of ethics committees when confronted by the sort of social changes encountered in IVF surrogacy? Various answers present themselves.

1. IVF surrogacy should never have been allowed into society. Only in this way can one stop ethical and social drift.
2. IVF surrogacy should be allowed without any ethical guidelines or oversight.
3. IVF surrogacy should be allowed within prescribed ethical guidelines, which should never change in response to changing social mores.
4. IVF surrogacy should be allowed within prescribed ethical guidelines, which will inevitably be modified in response to social and perhaps scientific pressures.

The New Zealand ethics committee dealing with assisted reproductive technologies adopted position 4, whether wittingly or unwittingly. Could it have done otherwise? No matter what answer we give to this question, the guidelines it has used have provided ethical constraint and have protected the vulnerable parties in IVF surrogacy. In the last analysis, this is perhaps all that can be asked of ethics committees or of regulatory frameworks, which are never in a position to predict the unpredictable.

A Theological Addendum

What light might theological thinking throw upon liberalising moves such as those just discussed, or like the shift in the spectrum from A to D on embryo research and ESCs? It is one thing to decry the shift, but what criteria do we apply when denouncing it? Indeed, should it be denounced?

The boundaries delineated by Christian morals are usually more conservative than those of many scientists and community groups, even though the biblical writers rarely speak explicitly on biomedical

D. Gareth Jones

issues. The two reproductive areas dealt with in this chapter show that barriers can be set up at the conservative end of both continua – opposition to embryo research and opposition to IVF surrogacy. The intention then is to prevent practices moving in an increasingly liberal direction, that is, by sliding down what may be regarded as a slippery slope. However, most societies do not set up barriers at these same places, since with varying restrictions they allow some embryo and ESC research and also IVF surrogacy. What contribution can Christian social responsibility make, especially for those serving on government ethics committees? We need to be aware of the following considerations.

The move within society to adopt more liberal attitudes on reproductive ethical matters is matched, to varying degrees, by a similar ethical shift on the part of many within the Christian community, which has become increasingly open to new developments within the biomedical sphere, even if some of these are still ardently debated among Christians. Theological discussion demonstrates a diversity of viewpoints, pointing to ongoing theological shifts in perspective. It appears that Christians, as well as others, are modifying their stances, alongside developments in science and changes in social attitudes.

Neither science nor theology operates in a cultural vacuum. The science undertaken today is not the same as that conducted in the 1950s; the technological sophistication is quite different, but so is the cultural context. Much the same can be said for theology, which at its best is rooted in its culture, critiquing it and speaking to it. The theological questions raised by embryo research and IVF surrogacy were unknown in the 1950s, with the result that innate opposition to these procedures may reflect an outmoded theological framework rather than a nuanced response to the ethical issues.

Nevertheless, many theological commentators find considerable solace in the slippery slope argument. The limitation of this approach for public debate is that it allows no room for manoeuvre: once a procedure or practice has moved past some identified ethical boundary it has already moved onto a slippery slope and into unacceptable territory. The challenge is to discern what it is about the slippery slope notion that serves as an important theological driver – or whether it has no such driver. This is an important consideration since, once the slippery slope argument has been adopted, theological commentary will adopt a largely negative tone in public debate.

I am concerned about this, since it seems to me that a theological perspective should ask important pastoral questions. Do the procedures help people in need? Are any groups of people disadvantaged through use of the procedures? What important moral values, if any, are being transgressed, and which ones are being upheld? These are core theological questions regardless of where one sits along any conservative–liberal or cautionary–permissive continuum. It is not any particular point on a continuum that is definitive, but the moral drivers that underlie the way in which the procedures are being applied. Consequently, an apparently liberal drift, in and of itself, should not be a matter for concern, unless its likely end result is that people are demeaned and relationships central to their humanity are destroyed.

This is where public theology comes into its own, assessing and weighing up the possibilities open to society. Its prophetic stance should warn society against expecting too much of any scientific or clinical procedures, none of which ushers in a new humanity. There are no perfect babies, either now or in the future; human existence is not disease-free and never will be; tragedy and suffering will continue to accompany us regardless of the sophistication of biomedical technologies. Alongside these emphases, public theology also has a role in underlining the positive spin-offs of biomedical developments in advancing human welfare. The blessings have been many, and for these we should be grateful. However, the task of theology is also to remind us that these blessings should flow to all peoples and not just those of selected parts of the world and selected parts of some communities. The public voice of theology is needed as we struggle to enunciate and adapt regulations that will serve as many as possible and not just the privileged few.

J. STEPHEN BELLAMY

Two Cheers for Public Consultations: But Where Have all the Ethics Gone?

Consider this statement by the House of Commons Science and Technology Committee:

> Public opinion plays a major part in forming Government policy, whatever the scientific advice.[1]

Is this statement good news or bad news? It sounds like good news that public consultations about new technologies contribute directly to the shaping of the law. Surely no government in a democratic society would be at all comfortable going ahead with innovative or contentious legislation without sufficient public support? Moreover, an appropriate regard for public opinion might prevent researchers, clinicians or politicians from pressing ahead and forcing the acceptance of a procedure in which they have a vested interest, whether for the enhancement of their own status or for more pecuniary reasons. Yet the statement could also be bad news, either if it implies that scientists are widely mistrusted or if it means that public foibles based on unwarranted fears or lack of understanding can hold back genuinely positive advances in health and healing. Neither is it good news if public opinion is only to be followed when a group of politicians or other experts think it convenient; nor if public consultations are no more than window-dressing exercises to make a government or committee look receptive to those whom they serve, while in fact camouflaging the real policy-making process – especially if that process is in the hands of a small number of influential people dedicated less to any

---

1   House of Commons Science and Technology Committee, *The Scientific Advisory System, Fourth Report* (London: The Stationery Office, 2001), para. 55. Available at: http://www.publications.parliament.uk/pa/cm20001/cmselect/cmsctech/257/25706.htm. Accessed 14 September 2006.

societal concerns than to ideas such as 'progress', profitability or the dogma of absolute personal autonomy.

The question of public involvement in discussion becomes very highly charged when the subject under consideration is the possible employment of new genetic technologies involving the selection and use of human IVF embryos. For this reason, I want to focus on how these technologies – particularly those entailing pre-implantation genetic diagnosis (PGD) and social sex selection – featured and were dealt with in two recent public consultation processes in the UK. The first of these is the HFEA's consultation, 'Choices and Boundaries',[2] on using PGD for inherited cancer conditions; the second is the process begun in the public consultation undertaken by the House of Commons Science and Technology Committee, entitled 'Human Reproductive Technologies and the Law', prior to their subsequent report,[3] which then shaped the Government's public consultation on the review of the Human Fertilisation and Embryology Act.[4] In examining these consultations I shall ask whether they have been successful in eliciting a genuinely 'public' response, and shall also ask how far the HFEA's and the Science and Technology Committee's resulting reports reflect the input that they received from the public.

This book owes much to Gareth Jones's valuable contribution to ethical debate. He has consistently advocated a thoughtful Christian position about the use of embryos, informed by his high view of scripture and by his belief that, in dilemmas not easily resolved from scripture, we need to think carefully about how God would have us proceed. In particular, he has championed the view that embryos are 'protectable beings',[5] whose use, though permissible in certain circumstances, must be carefully limited and regulated. It is thus

2   HFEA, *Choices and Boundaries* (London: HFEA, 2005).
3   House of Commons Science and Technology Committee, *Human Reproductive Technologies and the Law, Fifth Report of Session 2004–05*, 2 vols (London: The Stationery Office, 2005). Hereafter referred to as the 'STC Report'.
4   Government Response to the Report from the House of Commons Science and Technology Committee: Human Reproductive Technologies and the Law (London: The Stationery Office, 2005).
5   D. Gareth Jones, 'The Human Embryo: Between Oblivion and Meaningful Life', *Science and Christian Belief* 6, 1994, pp.3–19, p.16.

pertinent also to ask whether in these recent consultations there are
any signs to indicate that attitudes towards the use of embryos are
changing, either in public responses or in the statements by the committees involved. So, is Donald Bruce right to suggest that the Science
and Technology Committee (STC) Report reveals 'a libertarian agenda which is ethically naïve and out of touch with society'?[6] In a
similar vein, when Gerard Mannion asserts that the HFEA's partisan
presentation of its 'Choices and Boundaries' consultation prevents it
reflecting genuine honest opinion and instead leads to 'managed
public opinion' and that proper ethical scrutiny is being avoided, does
his claim stand up to scrutiny?[7]

     First, however, it is necessary to look at some general findings
about public consultations in the field of genetics. The Wellcome
Trust notes that opinion polls do not lend themselves to consideration
of complex topics. Rather, attempts to engage with the public are increasingly focused on working with smaller groups of participants and
attempting to consult with them in considerably more detail. The
Trust's own long-term consultation about gene therapy concluded that
it was difficult to get people's attention and that there was 'little in the
way of a ready-made audience for a debate about genetic intervention'.[8] Although it became evident that it would always be easier
to reach people with a particular interest in a given subject and that
'for complex issues the interested group may be quite small',[9] the
process they used, with its mixed strategy of information and discussion over an extended period, was very useful for those who were
prepared to take part. More strikingly, they found that the views of
individuals were not particularly stable. Even though the variation in

---

6   Donald Bruce, 'Commons Committee Embryo Report Ethically Naïve and
      Disturbing', SRTP Press Release, 24 March 2005, paragraph 1. Available at:
      http://www.srtp.org.uk/embryols3.htm. Accessed 6 October 2006.
      Bruce speaks for the Church of Scotland's Society, Religion and Technology
      Project (SRTP).
7   Gerard Mannion, 'Genetics and the Ethics of Community', *Heythrop Journal*,
      2006, pp.226–56, p.235.
8   Wellcome Trust, *Information and Attitudes: Consulting the Public about Bio-
      medical Science* (London: Wellcome Trust, 2005), p.9.
9   Ibid., p.11.

opinion from one poll to the next *looked* little changed, this completely masked the fact that, when given information and the time to
digest it, a good many people were switching their views – but almost
the same number as became more permissive became more restrictive,
leading to an apparently small overall shift of opinion. This volatility
of public opinion on fertility treatment and embryo research was also
noted by the HFEA in its evidence to the European Assisted Reproduction Consortium.[10] It also discovered considerable public mistrust,
in that 'only a quarter of people trust those "in charge of new developments" to act in society's interests, while a third do not'.[11]

'Choices and Boundaries' – The HFEA's Public Consultation on the Use of PGD to Select Embryos free from Inherited Susceptibility to Cancer

This consultation was launched in November 2005 and invited responses to six questions by 16 January 2006, from individuals or
groups. These questions asked about respondents' general views on
the acceptability of PGD; whether certain inherited cancer conditions
with less than full penetrance and with late onset constituted serious
genetic conditions or could be considered a significant risk; on how
much emphasis should be placed on the views of people seeking
treatment; whether the use of PGD should be consistent with current
practice in prenatal diagnosis; and what conditions should never be
tested for in embryos using PGD. The questions were presented in a
booklet which was freely available from the HFEA or downloadable
from their website. Replies could be sent online, by e-mail or by post.
    In addition, as a further part of the consultation, an afternoon

---

10   HFEA, Evidence to the European Assisted Conception Consortium, 22 July
     2005. See: http://www.hfea.gov.uk/cps/rde/xbcr/SID-3F57D79B-FBD 5B6BB/
     hfea/2005-01-07_FINAL_European_Consortium_EACC_public_attitudes_to.
     pdf, p.16. Accessed 14 September 2006.
11   Ibid., p.5.

open meeting was held at the Royal Society on 12 December 2005. This was attended by 118 people, the majority of whom were academics and people working in or with IVF centres. It was an enjoyable and informative afternoon, with several clear and helpful presentations from the platform, all of which put the positive case for making the changes which were up for consultation. I left the afternoon discussion in no doubt that the HFEA *would* go ahead and license PGD for the inherited cancer conditions being considered. Though I am indeed in favour of the acceptance, with caveats, of the new proposals, I was concerned that, at the afternoon discussion, it was obvious that the HFEA was in no sense neutral about the introduction of PGD for these conditions. Its members were not simply waiting for guidance from the public as to whether to proceed or not, rather they obviously *wanted* to be able to offer PGD for these conditions. Surely, though, any consultation that seeks genuinely to ask 'should we do this new thing?' is deficient unless there is a genuine debate, which needs to include a full discussion of the reasons why it might *not* be right to go ahead. In the case in question, these reasons are not merely about the utilitarian issue of safety but also address concerns for the proper use of embryos which, according to British law, are not to be considered devoid of moral status. The HFEA are well used to engaging in such a fair and broad style of debate, as shown by their excellent consultation event in Cardiff on 6 January 2006, which allowed 28 young people, aged from 16 to 19, to debate some of the issues described in 'Choices and Boundaries'.[12] A key feature of this event was that there were an equal number of presentations for and against the use of PGD to select embryos free from inherited susceptibilities to cancer. Interestingly, the movement of opinion amongst the 16–19-year-olds, shown by votes before and after the debate, was generally towards a more cautious attitude to using PGD for these conditions. One wonders why the 'Choices and Boundaries' consultation in London could not similarly have had contributions putting opposing sides of the argument.

12   See: http://www.wgp.cf.ac.uk/documents/HFEAResponseUoGTQWGP_000. pdf. Accessed 6 October 2006. In 2005, the HFEA worked with the Wellcome Trust to hold an innovative 3-day Citizens' Jury for twelve teenagers on the subject of 'Designer Babies'.

Perhaps it was felt that this would give too much credence to a view which might prevent the progress which the HFEA desired, or maybe it was realised that anyone speaking to the particular audience at that afternoon discussion would have had a hard job getting a contrary view across when the vast majority present – interested academics and health-related professionals – were sure it was right to proceed? Whatever the reason, conspicuously absent from the afternoon event was any debate about whether these conditions merited the formation and discard of IVF embryos. Utilitarian issues about risk, effectiveness, practicality and cost were the only things that counted. A couple of comments from people who would not use PGD even if they could were included in the consultation document, but there was no consideration of the ethics of embryo discard and selection entailed in PGD.

It is an acknowledged fact that it would be impossible for anyone who disagrees with embryo use and selection to be a member of the HFEA. The STC Report mentions this,[13] and the then Chair of the HFEA, Dame Suzi Leather, agreed that this was the case when interviewed by the STC.[14] Given that this means that a section of the public are neither eligible to sit on the HFEA nor effectively represented by them, it is doubly necessary that in a public consultation some room is given to dissenting viewpoints. Thus when, as in the 'Choices and Boundaries' afternoon, no arrangements are put in place for the case opposing the new proposals to be made from the platform, suspicions are aroused that the HFEA is not 'consulting' at all, but is merely presenting reasons to proceed. It could just be going through the motions to look as if genuine consultation is happening, in order to hide the fact that decisions about proceeding are all but made already.

Turning to the results of the HFEA's public consultation, two facts stand out clearly. Firstly, the very low response from the public: the total number of responses to the written public consultation was only 283. This bears eloquent testimony to the difficulty of galvanising public interest in these issues; doubly so when the questions, as in this consultation, are so complex. In analysing their respondents, the HFEA revealed that 156 of the 283, that is 56 per cent, were

---

13   STC Report, vol. 1, Recommendations 48 and 49, p.182.
14   Ibid., vol. 2, Ev. 177, Q.1259.

school pupils and that only 60 adults were 'unaffiliated' respondents, that is, having no professional involvement in PGD or attachment to a group with interests therein. While sympathising with the HFEA about the paucity of response after its laudable efforts in launching the consultation, we might also expect it to have expressed disappointment at such a low level of response. On the contrary, the HFEA considered that 'the public discussion was a valuable exercise in gauging true public opinion'![15] Moreover, it stated that a 'large number' of pupils had responded and that it was 'really pleased there was such strong interest in this by younger members of the public'. I would certainly agree that it is vital that young people are engaged by these discussions and that the teachers who encouraged their classes to make a response are to be congratulated, for without their pupils' replies there would have been only 127 responses. Yet, the HFEA's comments stretch credibility if they really invite us to believe that public opinion in the UK had truly been engaged with.

Secondly, there was a distinct divergence between the assured acceptance of the new use of PGD in the afternoon audience and the hugely equivocal response from the wider group of respondents to the written consultation.[16] As the HFEA notes, 'the meeting and the written responses represented quite different groups of stakeholders'.[17] The HFEA report on the consultation states that 'there was a significant proportion' of respondents who did not agree with using PGD for these inherited cancer susceptibilities. This group included those who disagreed with any use of PGD or felt that this particular extension of its use was inappropriate. The HFEA says that because the questions asked were 'open' and not limited to a range of specific, predetermined options, it did not think it appropriate to provide a numerical analysis of the responses received. Yet for all the openness of the subsequent questions, the first was eminently amenable to a

---

15   HFEA minutes of meeting of 10 May 20006, p.4. Available at: http://www.hfea.gov.uk/cps/rde/xbcr/ SID-3F57D79B-F8AF2A59/hfea/2006-06-14_Authority_minutes_MAY_10_05_06_314_final.pdf. Accessed 14 September 2006.
16   HFEA, *Choices and Boundaries Report* (London: HFEA, 2006).
17   Ibid., p.6.

straightforward analysis of public opinion, for it asked: 'Do you agree with the use of PGD in general?' The very fact that the HFEA noted that a significant proportion of replies opposed PGD reveals that it would have been very easy to give an overview of the acceptability of PGD according to this consultation. So why was this readily available information about the percentage for and against PGD in the public response not presented? Could it be that the figures would not only have shown that the respondents were far from unanimous, but maybe also that amongst those who were 'unaffiliated' there was a majority *against* PGD? Admitting to such a response and then, despite this, proceeding to allow the extension of PGD would appear to undermine the point of having undertaken a public consultation exercise in the first place. This is, of course, all merely speculation, but the HFEA could have allayed any such doubts by providing a numerical break-down of the responses relating to this question.

I agree with this extension of PGD, and I am a supporter of the HFEA (for the time being) and appreciate the work it does to regulate the use of IVF embryos in the UK. I am aware of how difficult it is to get people to discuss these complex issues and am not even convinced that the public always get things right, though there is evidence in some public discussions of a deeper moral sense and a higher level of caution than is exhibited by the HFEA.[18] Despite all this, the consultation leaves me uneasy because one thing is clear – what determined the final decision of the HFEA about the questions raised in 'Choices and Boundaries' was *not* public opinion. That may or may not be a bad thing; what is crucial is that we should not pretend that it was public opinion that finally did determine the outcome. It therefore follows that we have to ask what the basis was on which the HFEA did in fact make its decision to go ahead with this extension of PGD.

The answer may lie in the paper before the Authority when it met

---

18   Celia Deane-Drummond, Bronislaw Szerszynski and Robin Grove-White, 'Ge-
      netically Modified Theology: The Religious Dimensions of Public Concerns
      about Agricultural Biotechnology', in *Re-ordering Nature: Theology, Society
      and the New Genetics*, ed. Celia Deane-Drummond, Bronislaw Szerszynski and
      Robin Grove-White (London: T. & T. Clark, 2003), pp.17–38.

to make its decision.[19] This paper stated that, in coming to a judgement, the HFEA's members were to take into account four factors: (i) the features of the conditions themselves, (ii) the results of the public consultation, (iii) the recommendations of the Authority's Ethics and Law Committee (ELC), and (iv) the Authority's discussions on whether the conditions fit the current guidance for the use of PGD. But closer scrutiny of factors (i), (iii) and (iv) reveals that there is confusing duplication and that in effect there was only one input to set alongside the public consultation results. This is so because the first point – consideration of the features of the conditions – had already been included within (iii), in that the ELC had considered them and had concluded that the cancer susceptibilities are indeed serious genetic conditions. Not only that, but the first point is again covered in (iv), because the features of the conditions are spelt out again for the consideration of the Authority members. Thus conditions (i), (iii) and (iv) all combine to form just one factor – the combined judgement of the members of the HFEA's ELC and of the full HFEA itself. They made a judgement about whether the susceptibilities fit the guidance on conferring a significant risk of suffering a serious genetic condition. The Authority's paper had already noted that, because there was no public consensus on this issue, 'any Authority decision is unlikely to be welcomed by all groups'.[20] No clear direction had been given by the public consultation, and yet the HFEA made a decision to go ahead based on its own members' judgement – not that of the public – that the cancer susceptibilities in question did pose a significant risk of suffering a serious genetic condition.

Given that the public response was so equivocal, why did the HFEA go ahead? The fact that the HFEA was keen to gauge public opinion clearly did not mean that public hesitancy about proceeding would be allowed to hold up permission for extending PGD. Ultimately, the HFEA has the authority to make such a decision without regard to public opinion and, with many of the professionals it works

19   HFEA, Authority Paper, HFEA, 10 May 2006, 311. Available at: http://www. hfea.gov.uk/cps/rde/xbcr/SID-3F57D79B-4A29CF84/hfea/PGD_-_choices_and _boundaries.pdf. Accessed 6 October 2006.

20   Ibid., para. 4.4, p.5.

with pressing for acceptance, it is hard to see what could possibly have held the decision back. Relying on the authority vested in the HFEA might be all right if it were as balanced a body as possible (but, as we have noted, those people who do not approve of embryo use are effectively excluded from membership). Yet, after all, do we really believe that the public always gets it right?

The important point is that the HFEA should not give the impression that, in 'Choices and Boundaries', the views of the public had any effect on the outcome, except inasmuch as that public opinion was so divided that the HFEA decided to discount it and make its own mind up. Once that was the case, there was only one outcome that could possibly have ensued, but we are left wondering what level of public opposition would have been necessary for the HFEA to refrain from extending PGD to these new uses.

One final disappointing feature about this consultation was the brevity of the HFEA's report on it. Aside from being more open about the numbers who opposed the extension of PGD, the report could have been an extremely informative document if the HFEA had taken the opportunity to comment on the questions about the application of the new techniques in question that were raised by their respondents. For example, while the Church of England response gave a guarded acceptance of extending PGD to these conditions, it asked four significant questions which were worthy of a reply but which were ignored. These I shall now comment upon in turn.

1. 'Would PGD be used in this instance for a covert form of sex selection – such that a family's wish specifically for an unaffected *daughter* could be met (a case of the 'while you're at it' approach to PGD) – or would this be specifically disallowed so that the only test done was for the presence of the BRCA genes[21] irrespective of sex?'

This question is hugely important because, though I do not suggest this is necessarily the case, if the HFEA are planning to allow covert

---

21 BRCA genes are those which predispose the bearer to a much increased possibility of suffering breast or ovarian cancer.

sex selection when PGD for inherited breast cancers is used, then many people who initially agreed to its use would withdraw their support. The HFEA could have cleared this up by responding to the question, but the concern is that the issue has not even been discussed and that such sex selection might become a permitted, if hidden and undebated, feature of the use of PGD.

2. 'There is a serious lack of information regarding the long-term effects of PGD on children born after this procedure. What is the HFEA doing to ensure that this vital study is done?'

The question of the long-term safety of PGD was raised from the floor during the afternoon discussion of 12 December 2005. Though the need for such studies was admitted, as is frequently the case nothing was said about whether anyone was really going to do these studies and whether the HFEA was seriously pushing for them to be done.

3. 'There are questions about whether the stimulation of ovulation necessary for IVF is a particular danger to women with the BRCA 1 or BRCA 2 genes predisposing to breast/ovarian cancer. Will the HFEA investigate these dangers before allowing IVF and PGD to be done in women with the BRCA 1 or 2 genes?'

It would, in my view, be very helpful if the HFEA would clarify its position regarding this safety concern.

4. 'Will the HFEA continue to consult the public about any ex-tensions of PGD to other lower penetrance conditions?'

The HFEA could give an idea of how likely it is to need to consider further extensions of PGD to even lower penetrance conditions and whether such deliberations would ask for the views of the public.

The report on the consultation could certainly have included dis-cussion of these and other genuinely important questions which were raised by respondents but nowhere examined by the HFEA in the consultation exercise. Such a response would have helped dispel some of the doubts about how seriously the public's replies were being taken, as well as reassuring the questioners about the exact way the extension of PGD would be implemented.

The Chair of the HFEA has said that the HFEA has to take the view that the law represents society's views.[22] That this is the case leads me to consider another recent public consultation and the report that followed it, which was undertaken by those who are responsible for framing our laws.

'Human Reproductive Technologies and the Law' – The House of Commons Science and Technology Committee's Online Public Consultation and Report

Prior to the publication of the above report,[23] the Science and Technology Committee (STC) engaged in an online public consultation for eight weeks, beginning 22 January 2004, which elicited the views of the public on screening and therapy; surrogacy and donation; consent and confidentiality; and new fertility treatments. Sections devoted to human cloning and to general comments were also added. A total of 181 members of various organisations and 152 private individuals registered to take part in the online consultation, while 111 logged on in order to post messages. As a result, the STC felt that the online consultation had proved to be a valued source of views.[24] The STC also received oral evidence from 78 witnesses (including some of the contributors to the online consultation) and written evidence from 77 individuals and organisations. Their report was published in March 2005. The Government made their response,[25] using the report's re-

22   STC Report, vol. 2, Ev. 177, Q.1260.
23   See note 3.
24   STC Report, vol. 1, para. 5, p.5.
25   See note 4.

commendations as the basis of its public consultation on the review of the Human Fertilisation and Embryology Act.[26]

It is impossible here to comment upon all of the STC's 104 recommendations, but bearing in mind the STC's express assurance that 'people's views WILL make a difference' (original capitals),[27] it is revealing to examine two particular features of this report: first, the source and effect of its most controversial statement about social sex selection being acceptable and, second, the report's ethical approach, which was regarded as suspect by half of the STC's members, who disowned the final report.

The STC's acceptance of social sex selection

The online consultation presented a number of scenarios concerning the issue of sex selection – these included going abroad to have a child of the required sex; sex selection on the web; sex selection to obtain an heir; and sex selection to avoid disease. An examination of the postings by the public which mention social sex selection in response to these scenarios shows a substantial majority against it, in a ratio of ten to one. A much larger and more detailed consultation on the subject of sex selection was undertaken by the HFEA in 2003.[28] This concluded that 80 per cent of people in the UK did not want sex selection techniques to be made available for non-medical reasons.[29] As a result, the HFEA recommended continuing with the policy of only allowing sex selection in order to avoid serious sex-linked disorders. In addition to the STC's own online consultation and the HFEA's recent study which concurred in showing overwhelming

26 Department of Health, *Review of the Fertilisation and Embryology Act: A Public Consultation* (London: Department of Health, 2005).

27 See: http://www.tellparliament.net/scitech/the_inquiry. Accessed 6 October 2006.

28 HFEA, *Sex Selection: Options for Regulation* (London: HFEA, 2003).

29 HFEA, Press Release, 'HFEA Announces Recommendations on Sex Selection', 12 November 2003. Available at: http://www.hfea.gov.uk/cps/rde/xchg/SID-3F57D79B-4A29CF84/hfea/hs.xsl/1026.html. Accessed 6 October 2006.

public opposition to social sex selection, the STC noted that this result was confirmed by research conducted by Professor Tom Shakespeare.

Yet, remarkably, the STC's response in its report was that 'nevertheless, we do not see this as adequate grounds for prohibition' of social sex selection.[30] It seems that, in the STC's view, public opinion has to be overruled because it is not driven by the same ethical stance as that taken by the STC itself, which insists on having, in advance, factual evidence of harm to individuals and society if there is to be any restriction at all on the reproductive freedom of the individual to do what one likes with one's IVF embryos. Interestingly, the Government expressly repudiated the STC's ethical premise, noting that 'the potential harms that should be taken into account may not necessarily be susceptible to demonstration and evidence in advance'.[31] Moreover, the STC's commitment to a purely utilitarian ethic, based on unbridled procreative liberty except where there is demonstrable harm, is likely to be used as a means of disqualifying any Christian input to the debate on sex selection. A Christian response could be founded on avoiding the commodification of children by treating them as objects of the parental desire for a child of a particular sex. This simply would not count, because wrongs which distort the relationship of parent and child would never be demonstrable enough for the STC to admit their weight. A thoughtful comment by Dr Gareth Leyshon, made in the online consultation, illustrates the STC's error here:

> ... if we engage in a quest to legislate based on facts alone, we run into the problem that non-religious moral reasoning is based on the idea that reason can give us the right answer – itself a belief rather than a fact. The only facts available are about what is scientifically possible, not the values represented by allowing or withholding such possibilities.[32]

Surprisingly, the STC Report does appear to admit that the commodification objection does indeed have some merit in the debate about sex

---

30   STC Report, vol. 1, para. 142, p.64.
31   Government Response to STC Report, para. 6, p.6.
32   See: http://www.tellparliament.net/scitech/node/view/42?from=50&comments_
     per_page=10. Accessed 6 October 2006.

selection,[33] and the text is rather equivocal, mentioning that 'the use and destruction of embryos does raise ethical issues and there are grounds for caution'.[34] Yet, astonishingly, the final sentence of this section – no doubt the most quoted from the whole report, given the media attention it attracted – is that: 'On balance we find no adequate justification for prohibiting the use of sex selection for family balancing.'[35] It is pertinent to ask how that came to be the conclusion of a panel of ten MPs whose views on reproductive technology represented a wide spectrum. The answer is simple, and is found in the minutes of the STC's discussion on 14 March 2005.[36] This final sentence supporting sex selection was a late amendment proposed by Dr Evan Harris MP, on which only five committee members voted and which was passed on a vote of three to two. This makes a mockery of the STC's own complaint about the HFEA, made to its Chair, 'that the decisions you make are in proportion to who turns up to the meetings on the day'.[37] Thus, because three MPs out of a committee of ten voted to support social sex selection, it looked as though this was the considered result of the careful deliberation of our lawmakers. In fact this discussion took place without four committee members present because of the proximity of a general election. Further, one member proposed the use of the guillotine to restrict the time available for discussion, so that the report could come to publication before the election. The operation of the guillotine resulted in one member of the committee leaving before the final amendments were voted on, as he felt that his points could not now be adequately discussed[38] and, subsequently, half the committee dissented from the finished report.

The STC's affirmation of sex selection is deeply worrying because it illustrates how a very few powerful people, three out of a committee of ten, can wield disproportionate influence in the face of

---

33   STC Report, vol. 1, para. 141, p.64.
34   Ibid., para. 142, p.64.
35   Ibid.
36   Ibid., p.203.
37   Ibid., vol. 2, Ev. 181, Q.1282.
38   House of Commons Science and Technology Committee, Inquiry into Human Reproductive Technologies and the Law, Eighth Special Report of 2004–05, p.4.

overwhelming public antipathy to sex selection. It also reminds us that, just because a report comes from a House of Commons Select Committee, this does not mean that the decisive contributions have come from people who are somehow impartial or have considered the issues dispassionately and have no axe to grind. The proposer of the amendment about sex selection is an honorary member of the National Secular Society, who hail him as 'one of the most outspoken secularists in parliament'.[39] He is of course fully entitled to adopt as atheistic and militantly anti-Christian a stance as any other secular humanist might, and I strongly defend his right to do so. But we should not think for a moment that he therefore comes to issues like these without a deep emotional commitment to one particular viewpoint that may have disproportionately influenced the outcome of the report – an outcome with which five members not only disagreed but found to be incompatible with the STC's own ethical intentions as stated at the beginning of the report. As we shall see, the STC Report was internally inconsistent in its ethics and was unrepresentative of the STC's membership.

In its response to the STC Report, the Church of England's Mission and Public Affairs Council expressed concerns about the commodification of children. Its Vice-Chairman, Bishop Tom Butler, warned against regarding the child 'as an extension of parental consumer choice' as parents should 'not be led into believing that they can select children as they would a customised personal accessory'.[40] The Government response to the STC's acceptance of sex selection was disappointingly weak. Though it confirmed that it had no plans to alter its position to allow sex selection for social reasons, it agreed to ask for the 'public's views on whether sex selection for family balancing purposes should be permitted, as recommended by the Committee'.[41] Or rather, by three members of the committee! It is unclear

---

39   See the National Secular Society website at: http://www.secularism.org.uk/dr.evanharrismp.html?CPID=084bb6d445e81eb1414d9c6c2c181a71. Accessed 6 October 2006.

40   Church of England, 'Serious Questions over Science Report', 24 March 2005. http://www.cofe.anglican.org/news/pr3105.html. Accessed 9 April 2005.

41   Government Response to STC Report, para. 45, p.19.

why the Government should feel that such a poorly supported amendment, which deliberately ignored public opinion, merited further public consultation on this issue. In its own public consultation on the Review of the HFE Act, the Government nowhere informs the public that the STC Report was dissented from by half of the membership, nor that only three out of ten voted in favour of this particular recommendation. Thankfully, in the new bill updating the law on embryo use, sex selection for non-medical purposes remains prohibited.

Because the STC Report is unrepresentative of the Select Committee itself, let alone of public opinion, it is informative to discover the basis of the deep-seated objection by half of its members.

Why the STC Report's ethical approach was regarded as suspect by half of the STC

In the July 2006 House of Commons debate on the STC Report, the present STC Chairman, Phil Willis MP, paid tribute to the work of the Chairman when the report was produced, Dr Ian Gibson MP.[42] However, Willis's view that the rift in the Select Committee simply reflected the predictable divisions in society over these issues is a glossing over of the real reasons why half the members disowned the report.

The STC Report purports to hold the same, gradualist view of the embryo as did the Warnock Report and the HFE Act, considering it to be 'the most ethically sound and pragmatic solution'.[43] It even asserts that no-one who submitted opinions or was interviewed expressed the view that the embryo had no moral status at all[44] and goes so far as to quote with approval John Polkinghorne when he says that:

> The very early embryo is entitled to a deep moral respect because of its potential humanity, so that it is not just a speck of protoplasm that you can do

---

42   House of Commons Hansard, 3 July 2006, Column 528. Available at: http://www.publications.parliament.uk/pa/cm200506/cmhansrd/cm060703/debtext/60703-0723.htm#06070310000621. Accessed 4 October 2006.

43   STC Report, vol. 1, para. 28, p.16.

44   Ibid.

what you like with and then flush it down the sink, but it is not yet fully a human being.[45]

However, it appears that, whatever the supposed position on the status of the embryo set out at the beginning of the report, this has been ineffective in preventing conclusions which are typical of an extreme libertarian, procreative autonomy position. The report, had it been honest, would have admitted that it effectively ascribes to the embryo no moral status, or at least none that would ever be more significant than the expressed wishes of parents-to-be.

This is not simply my interpretation of the report, but concurs with the firmly presented objections of five of the ten members of the Select Committee who had input to it, and who ultimately dissociated themselves from it in a minority report.[46] In their statement, the five dissenting members said:

> Had all of us been able to have been at the final session, sadly, as it stands, we would have been forced to vote against adoption of the report. We believe this report is unbalanced, light on ethics, goes too far in the direction of dereg- ulation and is too dismissive of public opinion and much of the evidence. This report was always going to be controversial but to adopt an extreme libertarian approach from the start, on the basis that there was never going to be unanim- ity, was wrong. A thorough redrafting was needed, to put ethics and regulation back at the heart of all the conclusions, but this never happened. As a result, we have a report which stresses a gradualist approach up front and the importance of regulation. But then it goes on to recommend creation of hybrid animal– human embryos, unregulated creation of embryos for research and unregulated screening out of disorders in embryos for reproduction. Half the committee simply could not sign up to this.[47]

45   J. C. Polkinghorne, 'The Person, the Soul and Genetic Engineering', *Journal of Medical Ethics* 30, 2004, pp.593–97, p.594.

46   House of Commons Science and Technology Committee, Inquiry into Human Reproductive Technologies and the Law, Eighth Special Report of 2004–05, p.2.

47   Sarah Boseley, 'Ethics Row as Choosing Baby's Sex Splits MPs', *Guardian*, 24 March 2005. See: http://www.guardian.co.uk/uk_news/story/0,3604,1444427, 00.html. Accessed 4 October 2006. See also: <http://www.politics.co.uk/ issueoftheday/statement-from-science-and-technology-committee-dissenting- members-$367617$366843.htm. Accessed 6 October 2006.

Thus, this was not a disagreement which occurred because it is hard to get unanimity on such subjects. Rather the dissenters noted that it was the lack of consistency in the report's ethics which prevented their signature, together with its easy dismissal of both public opinion and much of the evidence that the STC received. The veracity of the dissenters' claim that too little weight was given to the views of the public and of those who gave written or oral evidence is confirmed by an analysis of the contributors' viewpoints, which was referred to in the speech made by Ann Winterton MP in the Commons debate in July 2006.[48]

Ruth Noble and two other postgraduate students made a general analysis of the ethical positions taken by the contributors to the consultation, whether online, written or at an oral evidence session. Participants were categorised according to the stances taken by Professors Savulescu (libertarian) and Campbell (conservative) during the oral evidence session of 13 October 2004. All of the pro-life contributions were listed under Campbell, even though clearly their ethical position is much further to the right than his.[49] Among examples given by Noble of these contributions were:

> Professor Savulescu: 'I think the 1990 Act should be liberalised to allow more experimentation and also wider use of assisted reproduction for non traditional uses.'
> Professor Campbell: 'I think we are always in a balance between the allowing of liberty and the protection of the vulnerable.' (He later included society as a whole as part of the balancing act.)[50]

It was discovered that 86.8 per cent of the people who posted online comments were of a Campbell perspective, 2.8 per cent of a Savulescu perspective, and 10.4 per cent were undecided. With respect to the written and oral evidence, there were 42 group responses, of which

48 House of Commons Hansard, 3 July 2006, Column 539. Available at: http://www.publications.parliament.uk/pa/cm200506/cmhansrd/cm060703/debtext/60703-0724.htm#06070310000643. Accessed 6 October 2006.

49 Ruth Noble, 'The Validity of the Science and Technology Report is Questionable', para. 4, http://www.bioethics.ac.uk/commentary/2005-06.shtml. Accessed 6 October 2006.

50 Ibid, paras. 5 and 6.

85.7 per cent were of a Campbell perspective, 2.3 per cent of a Savulescu perspective, and 11.9 per cent were inconclusive; while, of the 53 individuals who responded, 56.6 per cent were of a Campbell perspective, 26.4 per cent of a Savulescu perspective, and 17 per cent were inconclusive. Noble concluded that:

> These results clearly show the weight of evidence is in favour of maintaining the status quo and *not* changing significantly from the position in 1990. … [The STC Report] completely ignores the evidence and does not, therefore, accurately reflect the broader concerns of society. The protection for the embryo enshrined in the 1990 Act has been completely ignored; there is a clear bias in favour of libertarian minority opinions with continued references to John Harris, Julian Savulescu, Emily Jackson and others of similar beliefs; there is endorsement of social sex selection …; there are minimal rights for children; and the harm principle is limited exclusively to physical harms.[51]

Donald Bruce from the Church of Scotland's Society, Religion and Technology Project similarly criticised the STC Report. He identifies the report's shortcomings in implying that 'on highly sensitive issues like sex selection or cloning, risk is the only substantive issue at stake. Moral considerations are secondary or a regulatory nuisance'.[52] Bruce notes that a similar attitude prevailed when GM foods were introduced in the UK and the resulting public backlash 'unnecessarily lost what was once an important area of UK science'.[53]

It is indeed disturbing that the STC's stated commitment to a gradualist view, which implies a degree of protection and respect for the embryo, has been emptied of any such significance because the Select Committee have not allowed this view to place any meaningful restraints on embryo use. This is the corollary of accepting an ethic of unconstrained procreative liberty, which is out of touch with the majority in the UK as well as being completely unacceptable from a Christian perspective.

51   Ibid., para. 9.
52   Bruce, SRTP Press Release, para. 4.
53   Ibid.

The shortcomings of an unrestrained procreative liberty approach

John Robertson defined procreative liberty as 'the freedom either to have children or to avoid having them'.[54] The STC Report concurs with Robertson's assertion that the burden of proof rests with those who would restrict reproductive freedom[55] to show that what they would wish to prevent will cause 'substantial harm',[56] because this is the only acceptable reason for denying the primacy of the autonomous will. A Christian critique of procreative liberty will point out that the freedom it purports to bring translates easily into an enslavement to self. Greater choice does not necessarily lead to greater freedom, it more likely results in greater selfishness, for 'faced with a world of choice, our primitive selves want everything'.[57] As Cynthia Cohen and Mary Anderlik observe, the increase in choice that procreative liberty brings 'erodes the structures which give choice meaning'.[58] In particular, procreative liberty's stance on reproduction has 'minimal regard for the welfare of the women involved, the good of the resulting children, or the integrity of significant familial and social roles'.[59] Procreative liberty's rationalisation that 'if it hurts no-one else, I can do what I like' ignores the harm we do to ourselves if we live only to please ourselves. Yet it is widely held and sounds attractive in the liberal democracies of the West, for it seeks to prevent what is seen as unwarranted interference from the state and to uphold the ethos of the

---

54 John A. Robertson, *Children of Choice: Freedom and the New Reproductive Technologies* (Princeton: Princeton University Press, 1994), p.22.
55 STC Report, vol. 1, Recommendation 30, p.179.
56 Robertson, *Children of Choice,* p.24.
57 Gerard Rochford, 'The Allure of Choice and the Force of Destiny', in *The Christian Family: A Concept in Crisis,* ed. Hugh S. Pyper (Norwich: Canterbury Press, 1996), pp.118–29, p.119.
58 Cynthia B. Cohen and Mary R. Anderlik, 'Creating and Shaping Future Children', in *A Christian Response to the New Genetics: Religious, Ethical and Social Issues,* ed. David H. Smith and Cynthia B. Cohen (Oxford: Rowman and Littlefield, 2003), p.84.
59 Ibid.

individualistic, consumer-driven culture which is taken for granted in the West.

Robertson regards embryos as not having rights or interests – and this is sufficient for him to define embryos as lacking the necessary intrinsic moral status that would lead to any consideration of harm being done by their disposal. Rather, as those beings which have the potential to become human beings, they are granted only symbolic value, that is, non-intrinsic value.[60] This symbolic value is virtually devoid of moral weight because no appeal to it can overturn any use of the embryo that a potential parent, who already has interests and rights, might wish to make. Robertson also affirms that procreative liberty confers the right to have the *kind* of child the parents want, whether advantaged or disabled by their intervention. Understandably, Bonnie Steinbock remarks that: 'This is procreative liberty gone mad. Respecting the right to reproduce does not require us to facilitate the birth of children with horrendous, lethal diseases.'[61] In a similar vein, Thomas Murray concludes that procreative liberty 'prohibits or condemns almost nothing ... [and] has difficulty summoning the ethical will to curb the indulgence of almost any parental whim'.[62] Thus procreative liberty's lack of any consideration of the welfare of any child that might result from the use of IVF is a major ethical weakness.

An argument can be made from a Christian perspective that only embryo selections that do not distort the relationship of acceptance by parents of children-to-be are allowable. Taken together with the Christian mandate to heal, this suggests that embryo selection is acceptable when the parental requests for it are reactive to a serious medical need but unacceptable when parents attempt to commission a child having the specific characteristics of their choice.

---

60 Gene Outka, 'The Ethics of Human Stem Cell Research', in *God and the Embryo, Religious Voices on Stem Cells and Cloning*, ed. Brent Waters and Ron Cole-Turner (Washington: Georgetown University Press, 2003), pp.29–64, p.35.

61 Bonnie Steinbock, 'A Call for Ethical Boundaries in Assisted Reproduction', *Women's Health Issues* 6, 1996, pp.144–47, p.147.

62 Thomas H. Murray, 'What Are Families For?: Getting to an Ethics of Reproductive Technology', *Hastings Center Report* 32, 2002, pp.41–45, pp.42, 45.

Clearly the central inconsistency in the ethical approach of the STC Report was to pretend it held to the kind of gradualist view of the embryo proposed by the Warnock Report, which camouflaged its actually embracing a firm commitment to the primacy of procreative autonomy – a position which, by definition, robs the embryo of anything but a meaningless and easily dismissed 'symbolic' value. The danger is that bodies other than the STC, such as the HFEA and the HGC, have, consciously or otherwise, drifted or been diverted into assuming such a procreative liberty ethic. A Christian response will provide a rationale for maintaining the degree of dignity conferred on the embryo by the Warnock Report. This response is that, though not yet of the same moral status as a living human being, the IVF embryo has the potential to become someone made in the image of God. Because of the special relationship with God and with the human family that being in the image of God confers, IVF embryos are never to be considered worthless – 'not just a speck of protoplasm that you can do what you like with and then flush it down the sink'.[63] As Howard Marshall comments, 'the recognition of human beings as persons of inherent worth and dignity and not as mere things or disposable objects may rest ultimately upon the biblical doctrine of creation in the image of God.'[64]

Summary and Conclusions

Public consultations like the two that have been considered here will continue as part of a process of involvement deemed to be valuable in a liberal democracy. Yet, from the above discussion, there is little sense that public opinion will greatly affect the deliberations of those, relatively few in number, who actually frame our laws or apply them in practice. This is partly because it is difficult to get the public

63   See note 45.
64   I. Howard Marshall, *Beyond the Bible: Moving from Scripture to Theology* (Milton Keynes: Paternoster, 2004), p.47, n.13.

interested, in any great numbers, in engaging with complex scientific and ethical issues and partly because public responses can be both volatile and equivocal. The HFEA consultation, 'Choices and Boundaries', resulted in the HFEA making its own mind up after, reportedly, no clear lead was forthcoming from the public – though no figures about the public response were presented to substantiate this. The STC Report disregarded the thrust of the majority of public online contributions, as well as the evidence received orally and in written form from its selected witnesses. Indeed, in the STC's discussion of the role of the public,[65] they admit to having made no efforts to quantify the views submitted to them. In their negative conclusions about public consultation, they 'would caution about using the weight of response to determine the outcome of any policy review' and they state that 'surveys and opinion polls provide useful input to policy development, but are essentially anecdotal and represent the views of a self-selecting group of individuals; often activists'.[66] This last comment is somewhat ironic given the way in which an activist on the STC succeeded, with only half the committee voting, in securing a controversial amendment on sex selection. The report was deservedly disowned by half the members of the STC.

It is, quite reasonably, argued that the HFEA could not function if it allowed people with an absolutist view of the IVF embryo into membership. However, in order to ensure that people with such views are not marginalised, it is important for a range of views (however inconvenient) to be included on the platform at consultations, otherwise such exercises become presentations and not consultations at all. Indeed, when bodies such as the HFEA set up a consultation which deals with complex scientific developments and their ethical import, the consulting body should take the trouble to address the specific and legitimate concerns raised by their respondents (for one example the Church of England) about the details of the application of the new technique in question.

Examination of these recent public consultations has raised the concern that the status of the embryo as described in the Warnock

65   STC Report, vol. 1, paragraphs. 357–61.
66   Ibid., para. 361.

Report and the 1990 HFE Act is being tacitly or deliberately bypassed in public committees. The tenor of the STC's commitment to a virtually unrestricted procreative autonomy ethic rightly alarmed half its members, especially as its report purported to uphold the existing view of the embryo as described by the Warnock Report and the 1990 HFE Act. This suggests that any respect for the embryo strong enough to resist the extreme procreative liberty approach must be linked, as in Gareth Jones's reasoning, to its potential, in the right circumstances, to become a person made in the image of God.[67]

In particular, the STC's acceptance of social sex selection was asserted in the face of much contrary opinion from a wide range of witnesses who gave evidence to the Select Committee, and also despite the established (and admitted) fact that a large proportion of the public is against allowing such selection. The STC would no doubt have adduced public opinion as a factor in its decision if that opinion had been favourable to its own preferred conclusions. This reminds us that even though there are equivocal responses from the public, it continues to be essential that Christian individuals and groups do respond in such consultations. Surely it cannot be impossible, for example, for each Church of England diocese to hold at least one meeting about these issues and to hope that maybe five people from each diocese, with some informed knowledge of the issues, might make a response. If this had happened, there would have been 215 Anglican responses to the HFEA consultation. Churches should endeavour to educate clergy and congregations so that they can make informed decisions and contribute to the debate and to consultations, and might also influence wider public opinion by helping others think through the issues. This does not presuppose that all Christians will be of one mind on all aspects of every consultation. But it should mean that there is a moderating effect on the extreme procreative liberty approach which deals only in the rights of parents and denies the embryo any significance whatsoever – an approach which seems to hold sway in many committees which deliberate on these issues but is

---

67   D. Gareth Jones, *Designers of the Future: Who Should Make the Decisions?* (Oxford: Monarch, 2005); and D. Gareth Jones, *Valuing People: Human Value in a World of Medical Technology* (Carlisle: Paternoster Press, 1999).

far from the norm across the generality of public opinion, let alone Christian opinion.

It is also vital that 'religious voices' are not excluded by those, such as the STC, who try to establish as dogma the view that restraint can only be applied where there is 'demonstrable harm'. Whilst the Government is to be congratulated for rebutting this approach, it was remiss in not informing the public, when it undertook its consultation on the review of the HFE Act, of the compromised nature of the STC Report, disowned by half its membership.

A common theme in the two consultations considered was of there being a lack of unanimity or a divided public opinion. Yet in neither case did this lead to the exercise of a precautionary principle which might have waited for greater assurance about the need to embrace a controversial technique. On the contrary, recommendations were made that society should press ahead anyway with these more novel uses of genetic technology.

At the time of writing, the HFEA have just completed a major public consultation on the production of inter-species embryos.[68] In contrast to the 'Choices and Boundaries' consultation, this has engaged with the public far more comprehensively, using an online questionnaire, a telephone opinion poll, deliberative work in groups for a mixed audience of participants, and a 'Question Time' style evening consultation with a panel representing a range of views, of which I was privileged to be a member. That this was a far more effective method of gauging public opinion cannot be doubted, and one hopes that this pattern might be repeated in the future.

Unfortunately, this costly style of consultation was only made possible through a considerable grant from Sciencewise. Moreover, to my dismay, the open meeting of the HFEA which considered the results of the consultation spent very little time commenting on the detailed results of this extensive piece of work. This suggested that the public consultation had little effect on the HFEA's decision – an impression bolstered by the Authority's greater focus on clarifying

68   HFEA, *Hybrids and Chimeras: A report on the findings of the consultation* (London: HFEA/Sciencewise, 2007).

whether cytoplasmic hybrids could be considered human enough to fall under its remit than on the responses of the public.

Relatively small numbers of people will continue to make the crucial decisions about the use of IVF embryos. This suggests that it is vital to encourage informed Christians not to shy away from membership of key committees which consider the ethics of genetic intervention, such as the HFEA, its Ethics and Law Committee and the HGC – in this respect Gareth Jones is exemplary – and also to encourage the full engagement of Christian MPs with these issues.

It saddens me as a supporter of the HFEA and one who admires its excellent work to see that a utilitarian and procreative liberty ethic concerned only with cost and risk to patients is beginning to dominate its thinking, with diminishing consideration being given to the morality indicated by a gradualist view of the embryo. If such an attitude does take irrevocable hold, then more moderate Christian voices such as mine will no longer be able to champion the HFEA, but will be driven into the same camp as biblical fundamentalists and pro-life lobbyists.

GERARD MANNION

Horses and Carts:
Ethics, Legislation and Regulation

This chapter discusses the current situation in Britain regarding the ethical and legal regulation of advances in science and medicine – in particular, advances in genetic medicine. It seeks to make a case that, rather than the ethical horse drawing the legislative cart and, in turn, the legislative horse pulling the scientific cart (which was the closing plea of my chapter in Part Two of this volume), the opposite is all too often the case in both of these scenarios. The virtues of truthfulness and accountability have preoccupied much discussion in moral theology and Christian ethics of late, not least in relation to perceived failings in the church. Here one might hope to appropriate some of the collective wisdom to emerge from such debates and relate it to wider public life.

So great is the concern about the issues at stake that the chapter adopts a forthrightness of tone that I would usually seek to avoid. But, there are times when, in the interests of ethics and of truthfulness and accountability, such a tone is necessary,

Without wishing to over-generalise, and again not overlooking the enormous debates and contributions offered to the advancement of ethical attentiveness in these areas – as testified by other writings in this volume, particularly those by Stephen Bellamy and Gareth Jones – it remains the case that 'science' can often relentlessly race far ahead; and at times can appear to do so oblivious to, or at best reluctantly making polite noises towards, the ethical and social implications and consequences of its own developments. Indeed, it can often seem that science dictates to legislation. In turn, legislation then dictates to ethical bodies and seeks to loosen, often significantly so, the ethical constraints that should properly be placed upon public policy and developments in science, technology and medicine. Of course there are numerous consultations, including public ones, but there can often be flaws in how these are planned, facilitated, delivered and acted on. Economic and political expediency can interfere with the legislative process as well, so further undermining the ethical scrutiny of major developments.

Indeed, to be frank, one could argue that, in countries such as the UK, the genuine and sustained influence of ethics upon public policy and scientific developments is actually becoming less and less significant – and this despite the fact that there have never been more so-called 'ethics' committees and procedures. One reason for this can be seen in the way that ethics is actually perceived and taught across different sectors of the academic community. Surveys have shown that in courses in science, medicine, technology and law there is less concern with learning ethical theory – what ethics is all about and the nature and process of genuine ethical discernment – than there is with discussing practical scenarios and learning about the legislative constraints that impact upon these.[1]

In other words, in many professional degree programmes the focus could be said to be more about learning how to 'cover one's back' in any given situation. In courses in other subjects – philosophy, theology and some of the social sciences – there has traditionally been much more emphasis given to theory and to the study of the very nature of ethics and of what ethical concepts, language and practice actually entail. (Some years ago, it could be said that some of these courses paid so much attention to theory that they never allowed much time for reflection upon practice. But, in most cases, the explosion of attention to practical and applied aspects of ethics has meant that this criticism no longer applies.) Whilst this is not to idealise any particular discipline, it does perhaps lend further illumination to the overall discussions contained in this volume, if one observes that it is usually those trained in one of the disciplines latterly mentioned who would urge a more cautious and ethically sensitive approach to new scientific

---

1   Such conclusions can be drawn, for example, from surveys carried out under the auspices of the Philosophical and Religious Studies section of the UK Learning and Teaching Support Network (LTSN) in 2003.

and technological developments, rather than a more permissive legislative approach.

But, no doubt compounded by this confusion as to what ethics is and what impact it should have in certain areas of life, there is a second major reason why (genuine) ethics (in contrast to simply meeting statutory requirements to the bare minimum in order to cover one's back) is being perceived to be less important or effective. This second reason is that it can, at times, appear that a loose and often *ad hoc* 'coalition' has formed amongst particular interest groups, including government ministers and bodies, the scientific and medical communities, much of the media and, indeed, even many 'experts' in ethics as such. The main goal of this 'coalition', or at least (and perhaps more accurately) its main achievement, would appear to be to reduce to a bare minimum the actual ethical limitations placed upon scientific, medical, economic and even political objectives. This 'coalition' (regardless of if and when its aims and actions collectively come together in intentional forms or otherwise) has proved remarkably effective at manipulating public opinion, and indeed the opinion of legislators, in their favour. Truthfulness and genuine accountability, then, are issues that need to take centre stage in more of our debates in these areas than they currently do.

Let me offer one brief example. I ask you to picture, on the one hand, an animal rights activist and, on the other, an Oxford professor seeking to find a cure for Alzheimer's disease. I have no doubt that you will envision a rabid fanatic in the case of the former and a person of reasonable and honourable intentions in the case of the latter. You would not, I suspect, picture a deeply pious, pacifist and principled pensioner as the former, or a ruthlessly determined career academic bent on a Nobel prize and prepared to do anything to get it[2] in the case of the latter. Why, one must ask, would such very biased and widely counter-factual perceptions immediately spring to mind, given that there are, of course, examples of both scenarios, whether in regard to

---

2   Even inflicting totally futile and unnecessary suffering upon a primate by cutting away parts of its brain, if this is required in order to satisfy the relevant legislative bodies that testing has been carried out first on animals.

those defending animal rights or to those pursuing research of purported medical relevance?

Certainly, many scientists and numerous politicians have honest and noble intentions and laudable principles. They are as committed to truthfulness and accountability as the most moral-minded of other citizens. But, being also representative of the wider human societies in which they live, a significant number are just as prone to have selfish and manipulative tendencies, to be just as concerned with 'feathering their nests' and furthering their own careers at the expense of others, as are the rest of the population in general. And so they are prepared to play with the facts, to distort and misrepresent 'evidence' and even to lie and deceive, in order to achieve their goals. Why should moral debate pretend otherwise? Recent ethical and theological debates, certainly in Roman Catholic circles, have identified the need to be open about such careerist and wider human vices and failings amongst church leaders and ministers, particularly in the wake of the sexual abuse scandals. Here the failings in truthfulness and accountability, particularly with reference to the shockingly expedient and immoral manner in which the abuse scandals and offenders were dealt with over a number of decades, offer much food for thought with regard to areas of public life and practice.

But let us here restrict our concerns, in the main, to science and medicine. Just as in other areas of life, we need to become more aware of precisely how governments and scientists are extremely good at 'managing' and even manipulating the media and public opinion over ethical issues. For example, the need for greater funding or greater licence in certain areas of scientific and medical research and practice is frequently presented in epic, indeed heroic, terms. In any calendar year, if one were to count the number of potential 'cures' for debilitating and often life-threatening diseases that are trumpeted in the world media, I am confident that the total would reach three figures. And such 'flag waving', as in all aspects of scientific and medical research that become the focus of media attention, is usually ended by a statement along the lines that: 'Professor so-and-so states that the research is at an early stage and much more work needs to be done, for which much greater funding will be necessary. But the "potential benefits to society are enormous," he adds'. Recent studies, conducted by scientists themselves as well as by media experts, provide ample evidence of the prevalence of this type of reportage.

Now such stories may well be perfectly true in some cases. In the majority they are patently not − or I would not be balding still, and the oncology and cardiology departments of our local hospitals would not be bursting at the seams! I am not claiming that medical advances are seldom forthcoming from research. I am simply pointing out that the claims made about the importance and likely achievements of such research are, in numerous cases, overstated.

In relation to our primary subject matter here, we thus frequently see potentially 'miraculous' cures for debilitating diseases put forward as the reason for permitting and funding certain scientific and medical research and practices. Powerful and emotive real-life 'case studies' are portrayed to illustrate the potential benefits that will accrue 'only if' such legislation is passed or such funding is made available. So we see the case for allowing the selection of one embryo over another on the basis of sex (following PGD) being presented in the media in heart-rending terms. Allowing it, for example, would enable a little boy with a rare disease to benefit from his potential brother's bone marrow via a transplant. But these 'real-life scenarios' which we are presented with are frequently, in reality, rare and isolated cases.

Some might argue that this does not make them any less valid, but the first point in response is to note that such cases are presented as if the instances involved are much more widespread than they are; and so the techniques involved thereby appear to have much more wide-ranging application than in actual fact they have. Secondly, what such tactics achieve is that the legislative and permissive (in a literal and non-pejorative sense) door is pushed ajar. Even if that door is opened just a little, it is almost always the case that it is never again shut. Indeed, more often than not it is gradually pushed further and further open, so that what becomes legally and socially acceptable and permissible increases more and more − out of all proportion to the original plea for licence, and indeed sometimes contrary to both the spirit and the letter of that original bid.

This is not just pointing out the familiar 'slippery slope' arguments − it is a statement of factual consequence. The most obvious example here, of course, is the UK's 1967 Abortion Act. Regardless of whether one is for or against abortion, it is an undeniable fact that both the spirit and letter of the 1967 Act have been widely flouted and ignored, ever since it passed into law, so that by now abortion in the UK[3] is available more or less on demand and, as research indicates, often for social (one might even say 'lifestyle') reasons rather than medical ones.

Indeed, today, when one listens to certain members of the UK's Human Fertilisation and Embryology Authority, in particular the Chair, speaking in the media, they often appear to be evangelists for the cause of the scientific and medical community who wish to push back the frontiers of what is permissible ever more. But why should members of a *regulatory* body so frequently seek to make the case, in public, for applying the minimum of regulation?

Yet this does not let ethicists off the hook, either. In a broadcast interview just a few years ago, one expert in ethics who served on various regulatory committees seemed, at the very least, somewhat naive in his attitude towards scientific and medical researchers. He sought to portray them as universally sincere and well-intentioned persons who are always seeking to do the good. He spoke of the 'careful' fashion in which animal experiments were carried out when he visited laboratories, without stopping to reflect that such pro-cedures could very easily be 'staged' for a visit from a member of a regulatory body. Nor, even, did he comment upon the video and documentary evidence that cruel, barbaric, sordid and torturous abuses often do take place in such labs – practices which are not simply unethical but also illegal.

Indeed, while considering the subject of carts and horses, might it be worth pondering upon the implications of the fact that Baroness Mary Warnock, the philosopher who chaired the committee which produced the initial report that led to legislation on research into fertil-isation and embryology, has admitted that both she and many other members of her committee had no specialist knowledge of the scien-tific and medical research and procedures they were being asked to

3   Except in Northern Ireland.

report upon – they simply 'learnt on the job'.[4] Indeed, Warnock even states that she, along with others on the committee, 'sat at the feet' of the one member who seemed to have the most relevant knowledge, Anne McLaren. It would appear not to have crossed Warnock's mind that, as Head of the Mammalian Development Unit of the Medical Research Council, McLaren's 'teaching' of her fellow committee members might have been a little biased or, at least, that she had a conflict of interest. Added to this, of course, is the fact that committees can be notoriously poor ways of achieving anything at all meaningful, let alone ethical scrutiny or even consensus.

So, does all this not mean that Warnock's committee were open to all forms of biased persuasion and rhetoric from those who stood to gain from a more liberal set of conclusions being reached in the report than pertained in the then status quo? And is this not all the more the case with regard to ethics committees and regulatory bodies today? After all, scientific and, especially, medical researchers and practitioners are very persuasive in making their case – they are trained to be so and can often resort to employing rhetoric and highly emotive language in going about such business. They will also usually have had years of experience in drawing up and presenting hugely convincing bids for research funding. A committee of lay people, and even professionals whose expertise is in fields different from those they are being asked to pass judgement upon, could prove to be a relative 'pushover' to a body of academic peers and administrators responsible for awarding millions of pounds in research grants.

In short, when it comes to legislation and regulation, it appears that social and truly ethical concerns are all too frequently pushed into the background as other issues prevail. The default position is not, as it should be, to exercise caution in order that full investigations and deliberations might be carried out with regard to the ethical status, along with the implications and long-term consequences, of certain scientific and medical aims, intentions and practices. Rather, the default position in the UK is to do all that can be done to 'open the door', however slightly ajar, in order that a continued and sustained

4   Mary Warnock, *A Memoir: People and Places* (London: Duckworth, 2002), p.36.

case can subsequently be made for it to be opened further and further. The result of this is that crucial ethical debates are often left behind and eventually become jettisoned altogether, because the legislation and the science have moved way beyond the matters which those ethical debates sought to address. Science, not ethics, forces the pace of legislation.[5]

This is notwithstanding the debates which have taken place in the UK about many of the technologies in question. The important point here is that, despite these having involved ethicists, philosophers, church groups, human rights experts and representative groups, protests against the tide of regulative permissiveness have often proved too little too late, as scientific, medical and governmental opinion has advanced in a particular direction that appears to have left ethics very far behind. Hence, the effect of any ethical lobbying has often been limited and piecemeal.

So then, the sincerity and effectiveness of attention to ethical questions in current procedures is something that needs to be examined afresh. How genuinely ethical are the considerations and deliberations? How open to manipulation by parties with vested interests are such discussions? What are the long-term attitudinal and social effects of all this? Let us explore such questions a little more.

In relation to the ongoing developments in genetic science, a further complication presented itself in 2005. As the development and

---

5   Here, debates concerning the precautionary principle (where decisions are made through erring on the side of caution with regard to potential negative consequences of particular technologies) are obviously relevant. But a fundamental problem is that some of those who favour much more permissiveness in allowing certain genetic techniques to be developed and practised argue that it is unclear 'in which direction (if any) caution lies', John Harris, 'The Ethical use of Human Embryonic Stem Cells', chapter 12, in Justine Burley and John Harris, *A Companion to Genethics* (Oxford: Blackwell, 2004), p.161. In other words, how do we decide where to exercise caution – what pros and cons do we weight against one another? I might add that perhaps a more telling problem here concerns the often *consequentialistic* nature of the thinking behind many applications of the precautionary principle. Numerous ethical theorists have demonstrated the potential pitfalls that lurk behind consequentialist ethical reasoning (at least when applied in isolation from other methods and theories in ethics).

licensing of further technologies and forms of embryonic experimentation has continued apace,[6] the HFEA, under fire, it would appear, from all sides and undergoing a UK government review of its remit and purpose, began to utilise its numerous media contacts and its own website to launch a series of 'consultations' of the general public regarding the 'acceptable limits' of the application of PGD[7] to screen for conditions of 'low penetrance'.[8] This, in itself, might be deemed to be no bad thing; but the manner in which the HFEA has conducted the consultation, the partisan aspects of the methodology employed in carrying it out and, finally, the presupposition that this can genuinely reflect honest opinion rather than 'managed public opinion' all suggest that the entire process is highly flawed. Rather than being an instance where the ethical debates precede the scientific and legislative actions, once again we detect that the scientific and legislative communities have all too easily been able to avoid genuine ethical scrutiny.

Note, also, that the consultation process itself was couched in partisan and emotive terms – for example, one consultation asked members of the public whether testing at conception for conditions such as Alzheimer's should be permitted. It also asked about allowing tests for certain types of prostate cancer and brain disease. An earlier consultation asked: 'Should people be allowed to select embryos free from an inherited susceptibility to cancer?' In both cases the scientific prompting is misleading and the promised benefits open to question, and so members of the public are being prevented from making an *informed* contribution to the debate, unless they go to great lengths to seek out the information, evidence and alternative viewpoints to be found elsewhere. Of course, more pressing issues are raised in the documentation with which the HFEA supports the process, but the dice are loaded from the outset by its presumption of the rightness of

6   Particularly in the UK (but increasingly, also, in the USA and elsewhere).
7   The HFEA has argued (successfully) that such public consultation should also extend to numerous other issues, including the experimentation on human embryos.
8   Meaning that people have a low risk of developing such a condition, even if the gene which can lead to the condition in question is present.

embarking upon what is ultimately a utilitarian form of analysis (and a very crude one at that) and by its opening with emotive and biased questions which, as any researcher knows, can have an enormous impact upon the response.

On 10 November 2005, Suzi Leather, the then Chair of the HFEA, explained the purpose of the consultation by arguing that it was necessary to engage in such a process; her reason being that, just because a new scientific or medical technique is possible, it does not necessarily mean that it is publicly acceptable.[9] Yet, aside from the fact that this returns us to the parameters of the famous debate between Lord Devlin and H. L. A. Hart about the nature and origins of morality and its relationship to the formation of laws,[10] it also suggests that yet again the HFEA are proceeding in the wrong fashion, and this for two reasons in particular.

First, Leather's statement is focused in the wrong place: it would have been more reassuring if she had stated that 'just because something is publicly acceptable is does not mean that it is right'. The Government learned this to their cost, when (only the day before Leather's statement) they tried to force through anti-terror legislation which would enable suspects to be detained for up to 90 days without being charged or put on trial. Even though opinion polls showed that this would be publicly acceptable, and even though much of the tabloid press was actively promoting the legislation,[11] the Blair Government suffered their first ever humiliating defeat in the House of Commons. This demonstrated, thankfully, that many MPs were of the mind that just because many members of the public might find the

9   In an interview with BBC Radio 4, 10 November 2005.
10   These were the famous debates concerning 'the man on the Clapham omnibus'. See Basil Mitchell, *Law, Morality and Religion in a Secular Society* (Oxford: OUP, 1970.
11   *The Sun* (no doubt following Government briefings) carried an emotive picture of one of the victims of the 7 July London bombings alongside a headline recommending members of the British parliament to 'do their duty' and support the legislation.

detention of suspects for 90 days without charge acceptable, that did not make it right.[12]

And this leads us into the second point. Public opinion can easily be manipulated, as we have seen with reference to the 'coalition of persuaders' discussed earlier. Of course the public would swing behind 90 days detention without trial when such an effective media and governmental 'spin' campaign, resorting to all the devices of propaganda, was in operation. But the public have neither sufficient scientific knowledge nor, crucially, an adequate ethical grounding to make an informed decision on such matters. Most of the public used to think it acceptable to smoke in public places, just as their parents most likely believed that smoking did little lasting harm to health. But, as the links between smoking and cancer emerged and, later, moral debates about the acceptability of enforcing passive smoking upon others entered the public arena, perceptions changed.

The public can be open to persuasion. Even in the case of smoking, that aforementioned powerful 'coalition' has simply swung behind the anti-smoking lobby (it keeps public health costs down). Had they swung the other way, perhaps public opinion today would be different – witness the fluctuations on the issues of the environment and genetically modified food.

Thus the point again here is that the moral debates need to be had first, in order that the legislative and scientific communities, and of course the general public, have at their disposal not only the full range of facts but also a comprehensive body of moral insight when coming to make decisions on matters of ethical concern. If the HFEA continues to evade its true obligations and goes the way of much governmental practice of late – in seeking to shift responsibility for its deliberative function onto the general public – then it should be disbanded, as even Lord Winston, the fertility pioneer and specialist,

---

12   This calls to mind the famous objection to certain forms of utilitarianism, which examines the scenario of the ten people in a room, eight of whom are sadists. Allowing them to torture the remaining two would, indeed, bring about greatest utility or happiness for the majority, but that alone does not mean it would be morally right or acceptable.

has suggested.[13] But this should only be made to happen when plans for a more accountable and effective body of moral discernment are in place and ready to be implemented the moment that the HFEA ceases to exist. This is because shifting the focus onto the general public assumes them to possess a range of knowledge and moral discernment, as well as the time and opportunity, that most people leading busy lives simply do not have. Furthermore, to allow a situation in which there were no public body responsible for exercising the HFEA's primary duties would give scope for the most powerful, wealthy and organised interest groups to wield undue influence upon scientific development and legislation and to seek to persuade the public of their own opinions and thereby promote their own priorities. And, as we have seen, this would result in moral and ethical concerns being placed way down the list of priorities.[14]

Returning to our discussion of horses and carts, we might here gain much from reflecting upon the thoughts of John Habgood, the former Archbishop of York, who is literate both in ethics (theological and philosophical) and in science. He has pointed to three 'slippery slopes' which can often beset such legislative procedures. First, the scientific techniques themselves may become extended beyond their original scope of concern or field of application. Second is the legal slippery slope – Habgood also uses the 1967 Abortion Act as a prime example of this. Third, and perhaps of especial relevance to our concerns here, is the 'slippery slope' in social and psychological factors. Again referring to the Abortion Act as an example, Habgood states:

13 Lord Winston has gone so far as to question the very usefulness of the HFEA and therefore its existence. He called for the HFEA to be disbanded, albeit on ground of its incompetence, and spoke of how this hinders scientific advancement. 'Abolish Fertility Watchdog Says IVF Expert', *The Times*, 10 December 2004.

14 For example, if a scientist or government minister wishes to see a particular form of experimentation passed primarily out of economic or even personal career reasons, he/she has already by-passed moral considerations altogether. Should that person then be allowed to influence public debate on the experimentation? One cannot help but view the HEFA's turn to the public, in light of the criticism it has sustained recently and of the governmental review of its remit, as well as the Government's penchant in recent years for utilising 'public consultation' for political ends, with a degree of scepticism.

> The growth of abortion-mindedness in Britain in the wake of the Abortion Act illustrates how it is not so much technical innovation, but social familiarity, which has been responsible for changing public perceptions about what is ethically acceptable. Medicine, as currently practised, is not well adapted to assess the long-term social impact of new forms of intervention [in reproduction].[15]

The achievement of such social 'familiarity', I would add, must be attributed in no small measure to the immensely successful presentation of the case for permissive legislative made by various parties across Government, medicine and science, and so willingly taken on board by the media: new 'social orthodoxies' emerge. But Habgood helps focus our attention upon a most important feature of these debates – if not *the* most important – namely the social context (what I would call the 'communitarian implications') of such technological advances and legislative ethical failings and consequent legislative permissiveness. Here we are concerned with the new 'perfection mindedness' which prevails as a result of the developments discussed elsewhere in this volume. As Habgood stated, addressing the then planned legislation (since enacted) to allow sexual selection of embryos in IVF treatment:

> Individual cases can always appear to be justified, and individual needs met without immediate harm. It is the accumulation of cases, the growth of habits and attitudes, which gradually mould public perception of what is happening and what it means. The history of much well-meaning legislation points overwhelmingly to the strong likelihood that sex selection would in the long run bring consumerisation and consumerist attitudes right into the heart of one of the most awesome personal experiences in any human life.[16]

Further, just as we have conflicts between differing perceptions and constructs of what it is to be an individual human being, so equally do we have competing conceptions about what it is to be a person-in-community. Seeing that there are such social ontologies that are not simply competing but are actually in mutual opposition, what are the implications of this in relation to genetic science and medicine and, in turn, what is the impact of these upon our communities? And who should explore such issues? As Habgood states, medicine is 'not well

---

15   John Habgood, 'Test-tube Idolatry', *The Tablet*, 2 August 2003, p.6.
16   Ibid.

adapted' to assessing the social and psychological impact of its own developments, and there are profound existential and what he deems to be 'idolatrous' consequences that follow when the social context is ignored.

Again, none of this is to forget the many debates which did take place at that time. The point is that the voices which often tend to prevail in relation to these and other recent developments are those which subordinate the ethical and social concerns to scientific, governmental and, indeed, individual concerns.

Lest anyone fear there is religious bias at work here, we should also take note of the arguments of Hilary Rose, a sociologist, and Steven Rose, a biologist, who have suggested that, in the UK, secular criticism of certain scientific and medical developments has been 'stifled' because the ethical debates are often presented (not least by the scientists themselves) as being between the right-to-life religious lobby and rational scientists who really care for the right to have a baby. We live in one of the most secular countries in the world, so the reprotechnologists can be sure of eventually pushing any innovation through, despite the ethical debates.[17]

They also address the media 'spin' on scientific 'advances', stating that 'with each new extravagant claim, the capacity to shock is weakened', and further: 'Few share the belief that scientific progress automatically generates social progress.'[18] They make a plea for the serious press to exercise more responsibility here because 'Pages of sentimental press coverage following the self-dramatising activities of

17   Hilary Rose and Steven Rose, 'Playing God', *The Guardian*, 3 July 2003, p.25. Even such an esteemed scientist and medical practitioner in this field as Lord Winston (albeit one very much in favour of the advances under discussion here) has spoken out against the wisdom of scientists and medical practitioners exaggerating the actual and potential benefits of new technologies. This was when addressing the British Association for the Advancement of Science, at their meeting at Trinity College, Dublin in September 2005, 'Scientists Guilty of "hyping" the Benefits of Genetic Research', *The Independent*, 5 September 2005.

18   Hilary Rose and Steven Rose, 'Playing God'.

a tiny minority get in the way of thinking deeply about human genetics as one of the biggest challenges of the 21st century.'[19]

In November 2007 it was announced that scientists in Japan and Wisconsin had achieved a breakthrough by 'reprogramming' adult stem cells to produce induced pluripotent stem cells. Now, assuming the findings of this research have not been hyped-up to appear more significant and further advanced than is actually the case, one might here ask the question: why have some countries and certain members of the scientific community been so aggressive in their campaigns to allow and to receive public funding for embryonic stem cell research, when the potential of adult stem cell research was still being developed and had yet to be undermined by the claims of the advocates of embryonic stem cell research? Notwithstanding the many debates about the relative pros and cons of the different types of benefit they could respectively yield and in what timescale, the November 2007 breakthrough would appear to offer further evidence that embryonic stem cell research might eventually prove to have been neither necessary nor ultimately productive or even cost-effective, whether in economic, social or moral terms. Yet the opponents of embryonic stem cell research still face a hostile lobby whenever and wherever they raise their views, being lumped together with right-wing religious extremists and those who stand in the way of medical progress.

Indeed, the alternative techniques pursued so aggressively might eventually turn out to have themselves been the obstacles to achieving the desired medical benefits sought. Human cloning, the numerous moral quandaries involved in finding appropriate sources of human embryos for experimental use, as well as the many dilemmas and moral quandaries involved – not simply in 'harvesting' embryos, but also in procedures such as creating, cloning or forming hybrid embryos – could all turn out to have been diversions leading research

19 Their case is for a switch from the curative to the preventive end, so instead of working on such headline-catching reproductive innovations, Britain should 'put money into affordable high-quality childcare, so that women who wanted them could have their babies younger. We need a society that promotes reproductive health rather than expensive technological fixes.' Ibid.

down wrong avenues that did not eventually lead to the highly desirable medical achievements and consequent clinical treatments.

Why? Because the necessary ethical debates were not allowed to
take place, and informed ethical opinions and considerations were not
allowed to influence the discernment at work amongst legislators and
scientists to a sufficient extent, because other influences and motivating factors were at work and prevailed.

Just as the leadership of the Roman Catholic church has learnt, in
a very painful way in recent times, that its members must be much
better at literally practising what they preach, and just as numerous
commentators have demonstrated the need for more ethically attentive
and genuine processes of accountability in that church; so, too, can we
make a plea that greater truthfulness and accountability be allowed to
flourish in debates over advances in genetic science and legislation.
Many of the other contributions in this book have helped towards
making a cumulative case to this end. So, perhaps this further argument serves as a practical suggestion on how to actually make this
become reality. Hence, I summon my metaphor again and reiterate yet
once more: it remains my plea that the norm, the default in practice,
becomes that we place the ethical horse before the legislative cart and,
in turn, the legislative horse before the scientific cart.

R. JOHN ELFORD

Conclusion

Gareth Jones writes as a scientist and a practising Christian who sees ethics and theology as '… providing the ethos within which science is undertaken'. Here is an unequivocal invitation from a distinguished scientist who looks to ethics and theology for constructive help with the dilemmas posed by the science he practises. It is an invitation, moreover, which is made with the offer of collaborative assistance. This book is one response to that invitation. Readers will, of course, decide for themselves whether or not anything in the preceding pages constitutes such constructive help. Even if it does, it will have been nothing more than a contribution to important ongoing discussions. Achieving that is, perhaps, all that a volume like this can realistically aspire to. But has it achieved even that? In what follows I will suggest why I think it has. The emphasis on the personal here is important. The views I will now express are not ones which would necessarily be shared by all the contributors to the book.

First, it might help to clarify even further what the phrase 'ethics and theology' has meant in this discussion. It refers, of course, to Christian ethics and theology. The most important thing to say about this is that Christianity does not have a monopoly over either of the disciplines. All that it can do is to contribute to wider ethical and theological debates, to which believers in others religions as well as secularists of all kinds also contribute. However, the phrase has a particular resonance in the Christian tradition because the two terms are, as it were, two sides of a coin, just as they are in the Jewish tradition from which so much is drawn. The simple reason for this is that Jewish, Christian and Islamic monotheism is, strictly, ethical monotheism. Yahweh, God the Father and Allah are three names used in the three religions for the same righteous God. This is a God whom the Prophet Amos described as requiring '… justice [to] roll down like

waters. And righteousness like an ever flowing stream.' (Amos 5:24)
All this is centrally reflected in the Christian understanding of the
relationship between faith and behaviour. Christianity is just as much
about doing as it is about believing. This was so important to the
earliest Christian communities that they engendered a 'way' of living
which was widely commented upon, not least because it enabled ordinary unlearned people to aspire to virtue; and this has been of the
essence of Christian orthodoxy ever since. It is the sole reason why
Christians have always sought to engage in serious moral debate.
'Engage' here means, for these reasons, 'contribute to'.

Before we consider what Christian ethics can do and might claim
to have done, it will be helpful to be clear about what it cannot do.
Firstly, it cannot produce unanimity of view. In any given instance,
Christians will disagree with one another about the things they should
believe as much as they will also disagree about what they should do.
Some of them, invariably, try to overcome this uncomfortable fact by
shouting loudly at each other, but this is always to no avail. It is, in
fact, counterproductive of serious discussion. That is not to say that
there are not Christians who are principled about specific matters.
There obviously are, and they always deserve a careful hearing. They,
however, on their part are most heard when they recognise that not all
their fellow religionists share their convictions and that they are more
likely to prevail if they join in with them in ongoing dialogue. The
plain fact is that, this side of the Kingdom of God, there will never be
agreement among Christians about what to do in every instance of
moral perplexity, or come to that, in very many of them. All this has
to be acknowledged for the restriction that it manifestly is, whenever
Christians want to express their views and values to a wider world.

Gareth Jones, mischievously, asks whether or not Christian
theology is ever capable of fraud, in a sense analogous to scientific
fraud.[1] This cannot be let pass without comment – the answer is 'yes'.
Some Christians do commit what is tantamount to scientific fraud.
They do this whenever they claim that something is indubitably the
case when it manifestly is not. There are two groups who have arguably done just this throughout the centuries. Adherents of the first

1   This volume, p.101.

group claim that the Bible can deliver certainty on this or that issue, simply because its text, as the word of God, has final authority for all time and in all matters. Membership of this group is far from fixed. Some, usually called Biblical fundamentalists, consistently espouse this view; others do so eclectically, opting into this standpoint just whenever they want to claim some particular thing about what the Bible teaches. It is my impression that these 'occasional' fundamentalists seem to be the greater in number. For reasons explained in my earlier chapter, the Bible is not capable of being used in this way. It is a living record of the lives of faith lived by different people in different circumstances over a period of some two thousand years. It is, therefore, important for that reason alone. Using its texts to deliver a presumed certainty of opinion in this or that ethical dilemma is, to put it bluntly, fraudulent. Biblical fundamentalists are doing nothing less than claiming that something is the case when it clearly is not. In this sense they are as guilty of fraud as are scientists who do the same thing in their field.

The other group of theologians who can be similarly charged with fraud are those who claim that, whilst the Bible may not be able to deliver certainty, the church can. This, of course, is the claim for magisterial authority. It is most commonly associated with the Roman Catholic church, but many of the Protestant churches have made and still do make a similar assertion. The claim is manifestly invalid, and even fraudulent in the sense we are using that term here. From where, it might be asked, do the churches get such authority? The Roman Catholic church is well aware of the pertinence of this question and never fails to point out that it derives its authority by papal succession from the first pope, St Peter. Quite apart from the dubious historical nature of that claim, its track record does not exactly validate it: much of what the magisterium teaches is not accepted by devout Roman Catholics, let alone by others – its teaching on birth control being the most commonly cited contemporary example of this. However, just as the assertion that the Bible does not deliver certainty in specific cases does not invalidate the importance of the Bible in moral debate, the claim that the church cannot deliver moral certainty does not negate the importance of the contribution that the church can and does make in moral quest. The amazing 29 Encyclicals of Pope John Paul II are an illustration of this. One does not have to accept the most strident claims for magisterial authority to recognise that these are contributions of the highest order to earnest contemporary debate. Similarly, contemporary sensitive discussions about magisterial authority are often nuanced to the extent that they do make profound contributions to wider debate, as exemplified by Gerard Mannion's recent book.[2] It is argued there that the view that the magisterium should be based solely in Rome, from where directives are issued to the worldwide church, is a late nineteenth-century concept. Those who might wish to sustain this (historically recent) view should remember that, prior to that time, the magisterium was more generally understood to include all the bishops, theologians and church members. This earlier (and arguably more authentic) view sought a *sensus fidelium* and considered this to be crucial to the establishment of doctrine and practice.

So, some theologians do commit fraud, just as some scientists do. One does not have to look beyond their common humanity to discover at least some of the reasons for this. Scientists and theologians naturally want to do their best for their disciplines and for humankind – we should not be surprised when, in their endeavours to do so, their judgement occasionally gets carried away. As well as sharing a common humanity, scientists and theologians who commit fraud act in common in misrepresenting what is given. That the given should always be treated as sacrosanct is sufficient reason not to fall into this trap; and this is something that must be recognised by all, whether scientists, theologians (or indeed scholars in any field).

Whilst this reply to Gareth Jones's question about the possibility of theological fraud is, in part, couched in the same light-hearted vein as was the question, I have tried to make a serious point. Christian theology and ethics can no more deliver certainty in any particular instance than science can. This realisation alone is sufficient to enable practitioners in the two fields to work together, as has happened in the writing of this book. Without such collaboration, theologians all too often and all too readily shout scientists down and no dialogue can even begin, let alone bear fruit. In the context of medical ethics, those

2   Gerard Mannion, *Ecclesiology and Postmodernity* (Collegeville, Minn: Michael Glazier, 2007).

who shout 'no playing God' at the scientists are among the foremost of this kind.

With these caveats, we can now begin our final discussion proper. This will be to ask two questions: first, what can Christian theology and ethics potentially do in dialogue with medicine; and, second, what might actually have been done, in this respect, in this book?

For a start, Christian theology and ethics can sit down and listen. This might seem so obvious as not to need mention. We have already considered some of the reasons why some theologians are not prepared to do this. Another reason for not doing this is, quite simply, because it is a difficult thing to do. To begin with, there are serious difficulties with language. Much of the vocabulary of science is, of necessity, technical in the extreme. Learning how to listen is therefore a skill that theologians have to acquire and, as we have seen, it does not always come naturally to them. All this invariably makes for long and hard work that cannot be shirked if serious and meaningful dialogue is ever to take place.

Such difficulty in listening is exacerbated wherever, as here, the scientific narrative is itself incomplete and emerging. Scientists know some things, but they assuredly know that their knowledge is far from complete. Moreover, given the rapidly emerging nature of technological knowledge, to which Gareth Jones referred in the Introduction, scientists are as engaged in the learning process as anyone else.

The second thing that theologians can do is to help identify the issues at stake. Here they can begin to bring their expertise to bear. The reason for this is that the issues are never exclusively scientific ones. They contain many other factors which are associated with the notions of human wellbeing and its betterment. These run through the gamut of secular considerations, such as those of justice and the common good, to other factors which raise questions about the nature and purpose of human dignity, and even about its final end. The notion of human dignity is itself complicated by the fact that it often contains tensions between the competing claims of individual and collective dignity.

Something else that theologians can bring to the discussion is a knowledge of the working of moral theory in their own traditions, as well as a knowledge of how this fits into the wider picture of human-kind's quest for virtue. They also bring passion and commitment. This does not count for nothing, however rational we might like to think we are or should be. Humanity is mysterious and messy stuff and the passions are often of its essence. If passions are not recognised for what they are at this level of debate, they will certainly emerge as the discussion widens out to include public opinion.

So, moral problems are an admixture of fact, of human interest and engagement, and of moral theory. Christian theologians do well when they remember all this and help to bring it to bear in particular discussions. But there is more, much more, to what they can do. Put simply, they can shed the light of optimism on difficult circumstances. This is no small thing. Counsels of despair too often and too readily prevail in the face of difficult circumstances. The Christian view of life counters them with the belief that life is good, because it is God created, and because it has a greater end in God's sight: nothing less than a glory, in fact. This is powerful stuff. It purveys hope, counters despair and generates an endeavour which can carry things forward. Even more than this, Christian theology embraces an understanding of God's redemptive grace, which means that all things are possible for the good, regardless of evidence to the contrary.[3] When it achieves all this in the face of human suffering it is often at its most profound.

All this and more is taken up by Gerard Mannion in his discussion of what he calls 'theologically-informed ethics'. His focus is in the spirit of what I have just outlined. He wants to know what it is that theologians '… bring to the table'. He makes a good case for them being at the table in the first place. It is premised on the fact that their real work is abroad in the world, rather than something they do when huddled together. This might seem like an obvious point to make, but it is not. The reason for this is that some recent developments in the study of morality have emphasised the importance of its contextual-isation. These so-called 'virtue ethics' have stressed that agreement on value theory can only be attained by like-minded people who share like-minded views of the world. This is a view which is open to many different interpretations. Whilst some see it as confining morality to

3   See my *The Ethics of Uncertainty* (Oxford: Oneworld, 2000), chapter 7.

community life, others see its strength in the fact that it moves the discussion of morality away from seeking moral absolutes, thereby making it more attentive to the complexities of particular circumstances. This latter interpretation enables it to be more pluralist in its outlook. Mannion agrees with virtue ethics to the extent that he recognises the importance of churches as 'moral communities', within which Christian people learn how ethics is shaped and informed by the Christian story. But all that is prolegomenon to the tasks that then need to be performed. These are discovered in the wider world where, Mannion stresses, the work of Christian value theory has to begin in earnest. Amongst other things, this requires Christian value theory to move with the times. This is not a sell-out to modernity. It is, rather, the only way in which the Christian message can be incarnated, to use an important theological word, in the present time. Without this it is nothing. The Word, as the writer of St John's Gospel so formatively stressed, has 'become flesh'. Interdisciplinarity is the means whereby it achieves this in morality. In other words, it has to be abroad in the world, listening and responding to the best of its ability and, hopefully, responding by the grace of God. This has been the driving force behind much of the work of the World Council of Churches and of the Second Vatican Council. All this and more has been the outcome of a strident and continuing debate among Christian ethicists about the nature and purpose of their profession. Mannion charts much of this in interesting and important detail. Christian theologians have no right to offer themselves as being of service to others unless they can show that they have a professional understanding of why they do so which is commensurate to the professional understandings of those they seek to collaborate with. Only when they have achieved this can they even begin to aspire to making the richness of their traditions relevant to the wider community. This is the key to the contributions made by all the other theological contributors to this book. What they do, of course, is explore various aspects of this which are particularly relevant to the topic under discussion.

We have now briefly considered what Christian theology and ethics cannot do and what it potentially can. We are but left with the challenging task of trying to identify what, if anything, of this has been achieved in this volume.

Its writers cannot, surely, be accused of not listening. All the chapters are expressions of a dialogue begun in open goodwill and carried out in that spirit. So much of what can eventually be achieved in a study such as this depends on the quality and integrity of the shared understandings on which the dialogue is based. Needless to say, this can only happen if there is patience and sensitivity on all sides. As has been pointed out repeatedly, the work of Gareth Jones is exemplary in this respect. That, in itself, is a challenge to the theologians to reciprocate in kind. Others will have to decide whether or not anything of that has been achieved here.

A recurrent theme has been the recognition that the created order is, for whatever reason, imperfect. From the early centuries of the life of the church, Christians have disagreed about why this should be the case. Some claimed that the imperfection was deliberately intended by God so that humankind could strive towards its perfection. Others held that it had been created perfect, but that human sinfulness had caused the imperfection. Both views, however, maintained that, amid all this imperfection, God's providential care was always at hand. This belief prevailed until historically quite recently. There is no space here to describe the widespread demise of this doctrine of providence in modern theology; suffice it to say that, though it is still held by some believers and theologians, for the greater part a harder realism now prevails. It does so to the point that some theologians, as here, take as fact that human life is time-limited and that it will probably self-destruct by one means or another. If this is accepted, the question to ask is what do we do about it in the meantime? The answer must be: continue to do as much as we possibly can. This emphasis on continuance is important, because so much has already been achieved in every way, and particularly in the medical sciences, to improve the human lot. Longevity is now taken for granted, at least in developed societies, but it is a recent phenomenon, as also is the widespread, but sadly far from universal, amelioration of human suffering. All this has been addressed throughout. Indeed, we have tried to show that in Christian theology there is a profound understanding of what it means to recognise human beings as having been created in the divine image, and therefore bearing what has been powerfully described as an 'alien dignity'.[4] This places on us all the obligation to try and reflect in all that we do the love and creativity of the Creator. As we have also seen, we have to do this without the omniscience of the Creator. For this reason, caution must be exercised. Here scientists such as Gareth Jones and Christian theologians have much, indeed perhaps everything, in common. Neither party advocates anything other than the most modest of advances, and both want to keep even these under the closest scrutiny.

There is, of course, the danger that even one such modest advance might unleash a proverbial genie of undesirability. Precedents for this, such as the thalidomide tragedy, are invariably cited. However, to do nothing, out of fear, is not an option that Christian theology should even entertain. This is because theology is imbued with convictions about the goodness of creation and the human participation in the fulfilment of its purposes under God. Such convictions run all the way through the foregoing discussion. It is important to Gareth Jones when, as a biomedical scientist, he is confronted by those in need and there exists the possibility of ameliorating avoidable human suffering. Nowhere is the importance of conscience, and the need for it to discharge its pastoral obligations to others, more poignant. Ann Marie Mealey, in her chapter, shows why this has to be 'informed' conscience. This requires 'moral wisdom' of the highest order. It is interactive at all levels and cannot avoid the obligation to translate itself into action. Anything less would be tantamount to pastoral irresponsibility and even moral cowardice. Mealey emphasises the importance of what we might call the free conscience, which is unencumbered by constraint of ideology or insidious social control. She also stresses the need for this to be achieved at the point where tradition and innovation are held in dynamic tension. These are important points that are central to what this book sets out to achieve. They alone show just how creative, responsive and aware, in the widest senses, the Christian understanding of conscience both is and needs to be, in discussions of this kind. Anything less than this, as she concludes, amounts to a failure of spiritual obligation.

---

4   Cf. Helmut Thielicke, *The Ethics of Sex* (London: James Clarke, 1964), p.26.

Adam Hood's chapter begins at this point, where the free and informed conscience acknowledges its responsibilities in the face of pastoral need. Drawing on the once influential, but, sadly, now comparatively neglected, writings of the Scottish theologian John Oman, Hood argues that human autonomy is a key human good. The first thing that has to be eschewed is what we might describe as reactionary self-indulgence – and some Christians, as he points out, espouse theologies that are prone to this. Human autonomy, or courageous living as Oman referred to it, is of the essence of Christ's exemplary way of life. Oman's understanding of 'the natural' as the God-given place where this autonomy can be exercised is central to his argument, and the point to which Hood draws our attention. Enabling others to access that autonomy through PGD is a profound thing. The circumstances in which human autonomy flourishes are ever changing. Remembering this is important, because it enables us to understand the life of faith as one which lives with the excitement of constant challenge. This precludes its being lived in the safe haven of self-comfort when all the indications are that the storm outside is the place to be. Indeed, it is Oman's point that there is no refuge from such natural storms, and that our true spiritual selves can only be found in the midst of them. All this is the melee of human experience in which the supernatural and the natural interact. It has no inherent stability, and this is the reason why human life understood in this way is enhanced by its also being understood as the life of faith. Awe and curiosity are of its very essence. What we call 'the natural' is not a once and for all given; it is but the name we use for our collected perceptions at any one time. The constant interaction of the supernatural with the natural lies behind the similarly constant progressive divine revelation in human affairs. Hood's expression of this, within which he quotes directly from Oman, is worth repeating. 'It is as people live in the light of the ideal here and now that they discover an "intercourse with a greatness which admits no finality, but requires absoluteness of loyalty both in seeking to know and to serve its ever expanding requirements".'[5] All of this, Hood concludes, requires flexibility and openness, scientific integrity and, again, human autonomy.

5   This volume, pp.67–68.

In my own discussion of divine human love and creativity, in Mannion's account of theologically-informed ethics, in Mealey's analysis of conscience, and in Hood's excursus into the relevance of Oman's understanding of the natural and the supernatural, this book attempts to get as close as possible to an account of what Jones calls the ethos of the Christian faith. It is one which is centrally mindful of what human beings can and cannot do, of the prowess of their scientific ingenuity and of their obligations to one another, which are understood as being given by God their Creator. (This is not an understanding of the life of faith that would be shared by those who see it as providing what is now called, in common parlance, a life lived in the 'comfort zone' of disengagement from the real challenges of contemporary living.) None of this, of course, solves the problems of bioethics at a stroke, but come to that neither does anything else. What, we might modestly claim, however, is that what it does is provide the ethos which Jones the scientist expects as Jones the Christian. At the very least it shows why there is nothing to be taken for granted, everything to be achieved, and every humility and caution to be exercised in doing so.

There is one aspect to this discussion which was deemed so important as to merit a complete section in the book. This is the issue of regulation. So much of the foregoing has recognised the importance, even the imperative, of making such cautious advances as can be carefully evaluated and monitored. Moreover, it has been recognised throughout that these things cannot be achieved by medicine, or even theology, alone. They embrace and must be answerable to informed public opinion. This is easy enough to acknowledge, but far from easy to realise. Stephen Bellamy's chapter shows why. It well illustrates the realities and practicalities entailed. Harnessing informed public opinion in the service of a greater good must not be avoided, but the nature of the harness is dependent in part upon public opinion itself. Our political structures and systems are clearly inadequate when it comes to processes for marshalling public consultation, let alone when it is necessary to legislate for an unknown future. Bellamy illustrates the reasons for this in his detailed analysis of two recent public consultations, one undertaken by the Human Fertilisation and Embryology Authority, the other by the House of Commons Science and

Technology Committee. His revelations here are startling. They show just how public opinion is 'managed' rather than gathered, and how poor the overall response rate is in such consultations. All this makes it difficult for someone like Bellamy, who wants to make reasonable progress with the issues, to find the all important *via media*. Only by this means can two undesirable extremes be avoided. The first is that of doing nothing, or of Luddism, which is certainly not an option for serious and morally motivated people, particularly Christians. The second is that of allowing anything. The obvious danger here is that to which Mannion draws attention. It is that of allowing the science to lead, dictate and even circumscribe public opinion. This, of course, is not a phenomenon which is limited to medical technology and ethics. It is endemic in technological societies and has been flagged up by novelists, such as Orwell, ever since recognitions about the nature of technology-led futures began to dawn. Technology, for reasons we have considered, is not, nor can it ever become, inherently virtuous. Of its nature it is morally neutral. Only its morally earnest users can even hope to reap its benefits and avoid its dangers. This is where the institutions of our liberal democracies are strained to their limits. Gareth Jones illustrates this in his overview of how some countries are dealing with PGD technology, while Bellamy notes how, in the UK, discussions are becoming focused on a procreative technology ethic which avoids all consideration of any limit to the use of IVF embryos.

The recognition of the need for regulation in this area of modern science, and of the scarce adequacy of the institutions with the responsibility to deliver it, is one salutary outcome of this discussion. It shows just how PGD technology raises political as well as more narrowly identifiable moral problems. It shows, also, why this is a much wider problem in those societies seeking to benefit from technology and not to be burdened by it.

Another important aspect of the discussion has been to draw attention to the distinction between the use of PGD and related technologies to treat disorders and diseases, particularly hereditary ones, and its use to enhance the human condition. Gareth Jones notes the concern that some contemporary Christian theologians have about the possible implications of using PGD to enhance the human state to a point where humans become transhuman. This, they argue, is the ultimate impiety and the point at which humans overstep the God-given limitations of their humanity. The spectre of large-scale programmes of human modification, such as those initiated by the Nazis, is invariably evoked at this point. All but the ideologically driven would, surely, baulk at this. Its implication that some human beings have less worth than others is nothing less than horrendous. If taken seriously for long enough by enough people, it would proffer the prospect of social engineering of an unspeakable dimension. Theologians who point this out are saying something crucially important. In doing so, however, are they right to conclude that no enhancement should ever be tolerated under any circumstances? Jones begins his reply to this question by asking what, precisely, enhancement is. In what he designates category 1,[6] it could entail nothing more than some human persons being made 'super-healthy' to a level that does not go beyond that attained by others who had not been 'enhanced' at all. Such people would not, therefore, stand out, or be at all different from their unenhanced fellows. Like them, they would be vulnerable to other diseases and be equally subject to the vagaries of the normal ageing processes. Changes brought about by such processes, as Jones points out, are already both widespread and accepted. Theological opposition to enhancement at this level would appear to be against common sense. The benefits to humankind have been, and potentially are, so great that it would be both churlish and lacking in humanity to resist them. Likewise, enhancement which sought but marginally to improve human performance in one specific aspect or another might not be unacceptable. These so-improved human beings could well be outperformed by 'unimproved' others. Again, this might be thought to be very little different from what already happens in high performing human activities such as athletics. To go beyond this, however, would clearly be to overstep a mark into the creation of a transhuman. Here the theological concerns noted earlier would be very relevant, and disapprobation would be called for. In drawing attention to these distinctions, Jones is making an important point. It is that the borderline between therapy and enhancement is not a clear one. His view is that we need to work with paradigms which leave room for such unclear

6   This volume, p.130.

borderlines and then go on to promote precise and serious ethical discussions that aim to refine our response to them.

Nothing in this book has been said that would gainsay this view. On the contrary, enough has been said to show why theologians and others should be very reticent about contesting this stance. Careful distinctions are of the essence of philosophical clarification. The purposes they can serve are of immense importance. In making fine distinctions in the context of the debate about the moral acceptability or otherwise of emerging practices in the medical sciences, Jones, as a scientist, is providing a crucial service to those who seek morally to evaluate what the sciences should or should not do. Whilst, of course, theology is not a necessary prerequisite for any such evaluation, what theologians might, it is hoped, have achieved in this volume is to point out the unacceptability of any theology that does not give proper heed to such subtle distinctions. Such theology is, to say the least, presumptuous in its claim to have understood the issues at stake. It is also less than honest in its endeavour to treat the natural world around us with the respect it deserves as something God-given and inherently good, despite its imperfections. Indeed, enough has been said throughout this volume to give us good reason to believe that it is because of these very imperfections that we should strive to do whatever we can about them. There will, of course, be limits to these strivings, and they will be best understood as moral limits. This is the very reason why no such exercise should ever be undertaken without an awareness of the limits. That awareness is of the essence of responsibly being human. Readers will decide for themselves whether this book has made some contribution to that end in this important area of scientific enquiry.

Notes on Contributors

J. STEPHEN BELLAMY is Vicar of St Nicholas Church, Durham.

R. JOHN ELFORD is Visiting Professor of Ethics at Leeds Metropolitan University.

ADAM HOOD is a Church of Scotland Minister and is Vice-Principal and Director of Research at the Queen's Foundation for Ecumenical Theological Education, Birmingham.

D. GARETH JONES is Deputy Vice-Chancellor (Academic and International) at the University of Otago, Dunedin, New Zealand, where he is also Professor of Anatomy and Structural Biology. He is Visiting Professor at Liverpool Hope University.

GERARD MANNION is the Chair of the Ecclesiological Investigations International Research Network and Director of the Centre for Study of Contemporary Ecclesiology.

ANN MARIE MEALEY is a Lecturer in Moral Theology at Trinity and All Saints University College, Leeds.

MAJA I. WHITAKER is an Assistant Research Fellow at the University of Otago, Dunedin, New Zealand.

General Index

Index of Names

New International Studies in Applied Ethics

SERIES EDITOR

Professor R. John Elford, Leeds Metropolitan University

New International Studies in Applied Ethics is a series based at Leeds Metropolitan University and associated with Virginia Theological Seminary. The series examines the ethical implications of selected areas of public life and concern. Subjects considered will include, but are not limited to, medicine, peace studies, international sport and higher education.

The series aims to publish volumes which are clearly written with a general academic readership in mind. Individual volumes may also be useful to those confronted with the issues discussed in their daily lives. A consistent emphasis is on recent developments in the subjects discussed and this is achieved by publishing volumes by writers who are foremost in their fields, as well as those with emerging reputations. Both secular and religious ethical views may be discussed as appropriate. No point of view is considered off-limits and controversy is not avoided.

The series includes both edited volumes and single-authored monographs. Submissions are welcome from all scholars in the field and should be addressed to either the series editor or the publisher.

Vol. 1   R. John Elford and D. Gareth Jones (eds)
          A Tangled Web: Medicine and Theology in Dialogue
          288 pages. 2009.
          ISBN: 978-3-03911-541-9